NATIVE AMERICAN
HERBALIST'S BIBLE

20 BOOKS IN 1

THE #1 OFFICIAL NATIVE HERBAL MEDICINE ENCYCLOPEDIA.500+ HERBAL MEDICINES & PLANT REMEDIES TO GROW IN YOUR PERSONAL GARDEN.

AYASHE CHAKWAINA

ABOUT THE AUTHOR

Ayashe Hatathly is a product of one of the oldest prehistoric residents of the northwestern plains: the Blackfeet Tribe. With history dating back over 13,000 years, his ancestors have passed down some of North America's most colorful traditions and ways of life.

Growing up, Ayashe witnessed how other tribe members celebrated ancient Native American rituals. These experiences created a sense of pride in him that he still carries today. His fondest memories are those shared with his grandparents — prominent tribal members who always pushed for the preservation of Blackfeet herbal healing practices.

One particular incident that has always stuck with Ayashe was when his grandfather gave him "snakeroot" to put in his boots to prevent rattlesnakes from biting him. His grandfather also told him to rub it around his room to avoid unwelcomed nightly visitors and to chew on it to effectively relieve colds and flu.

This sparked Ayashe's life-long fascination with the medicinal properties of Native American herbs. He pursued a degree in Native American Studies at the University of California-Berkeley, specializing in Native American medicine.

Today, Ayashe is an author and sought-after research consultant for farming and pharmaceutical companies that want to harness the benefits of Native American herbs. To say that he loves his job is an understatement. Not only is he helping build awareness for his people's traditions and culture, he is also creating opportunities to be closer to nature and giving back to the land that nurtured him and his ancestors.

When he's not working, Ayashe spends his days hiking, camping, and advocating for Native American rights throughout the United States. He also spends productive weekends writing books on Native American medicine, including his current bestseller *Native American Herbalist Bible.*

TABLE OF CONTENTS

Chapter 2: How to Prepare Herbal Medications 71

BOOK 3: NATIVE AMERICAN HERBAL REMEDIES 75

Chapter 1: Importance of Incorporating Herbs into Regular Diet 76

Chapter 2: Popular Herbal Native American Herbs & their Corresponding Remedies 84

BOOK 4: NATIVE AMERICAN HERBAL RECIPES 91

Chapter 1: Equipment Needed to Extract & Process Herbs...... 92

BOOK 5: HOW TO HANDLE AND STORE HERBAL EXTRACT 99

BOOK 6: BEST NATIVE AMERICAN HERBAL RECIPE 103

BOOK 14: HERBAL TERMINOLOGY FOR BEGINNERS 191

Chapter 1: Effective and Safe Use of Herbs 192

BOOK 15: THE LOST BOOK OF ASTRAL HERBS 197

Chapter 1: Native American Astral Herbs & their Use 198

BOOK 17: HERBAL MEDICINES & PLANT REMEDIES. -VOLUME 1.............225

BOOK 18: HERBAL MEDICINES & PLANT REMEDIES. -VOLUME 2 245

BOOK 19: HERBAL MEDICINES & PLANT REMEDIES. -VOLUME 3 263

BOOK 20: HERBAL MEDICINES & PLANT REMEDIES. -VOLUME 4 283

FREQUENTLY ASKED QUESTIONS...................................298

CONCLUSION...300

BONUS: VIDEO TUTORIAL...301

BOOK 1

NATIVE AMERICAN HERBAL ENCYCLOPEDIA

CHAPTER 1

BENEFITS OF HERBAL OVER MODERN MEDICINE

Herbal medicine is a type of medicine extracted from plant leaves, roots, seeds, and other parts of natural plants, and then administered in its natural form. On the other hand, modern medicine is a type of medicine manufactured by pharmaceutical firms for use in conventional hospitals.

Today, the benefits of herbal medicine have become so evident that even modern doctors appreciate their role in enhancing human health. In short, unlike years ago when a person had to choose one over the other, it is now generally accepted that you can rely on herbal medicine to improve and maintain your health without denying the unique role modern medicine plays.

For example, a person who dislocates his/her leg while walking can have the affected joint readjusted in a hospital setup, and then rely on herbal medicine to numb the pain and to hasten the healing process.

Owing to the popularity of herbal medicines, modern scientists have found a way of incorporating them into their modern practice.

It is also a fact that many of the so-called modern medications are extracted from natural plants, but then are taken through some kind of mechanical processes for formulation and preservation. In short, herbal medicines that many cultures have traditionally relied upon have today been embraced with renewed interest.

Overall, herbal medicines, as Native Americans discovered ages ago, have great health benefits that include the prolonging of human life.

Mitigated Side-Effects, Cost-Effectiveness, Wholesomeness, Empowerment & Preventive Capacity

Lack of side-effects is a big advantage of herbal extracts. Cost-effectiveness is another, and wholesomeness of herbal products is yet another. It is also advantageous that consumers of natural extracts feel empowered, but it is even more beneficial when you use herbal products with a capacity to prevent disease.

Minimal Side Effects

Among the benefits of herbal medicines is that side effects are minimal. The fact that they are administered in their natural form means the body responds to them favourably in the same way it responds to vegetables, fruits and other natural foods.

It is for that reason people on prescription medications are advised to consider replacing them with herbal medications.

Cost-effectiveness

Unlike prescription medicines, herbal medications are relatively cheaper. One reason herbal medications are easily affordable is the processes of producing them are simple and inexpensive.

At the same time, those who understand the use of herbal medications also adopt healthy living styles to mimic the traditional ways people depended on to remain fit. In the process, any ailments associated with modern medicines are avoided.

Herbal Treatments are Wholesome

Herbal medications, as you will see in later chapters of this book, are wholesome. The Native Americans, from whom a lot of these treatments are inherited, believed that as you try to heal the body, you will also heal your spirit. At the end of the day, you not only become physically fit, but also get mentally healthy.

Self-empowering

When using herbal medications, you are in control of the treatment process. This is unlike the use of modern medicines where the treatment process is dependent on your doctor and the conventional scientific process.

Although there is guidance on how to use herbal medications, traditional healers primarily educate the people interested in using them and then leave the individuals to use what they want.

Preventive Capacity

Herbal medications are mainly recommended for the purposes of preventing disease, unlike modern treatments that are mainly used to treat disease. Prevention is certainly better than a cure, and so herbal medications can sustain health better. Herbal medications are even more preferable when you consider that many of the modern medications prescribed end up suppressing disease symptoms rather than eliminating the root cause.

Herbal extracts are rich in vitamins and antibodies, as well as minerals and other beneficial elements. They are, therefore, effective in strengthening the health of the body, and more so the immune system.

In fact, because they are great at enhancing the digestive function, those who regularly consume herbal extracts have a healthy gut. This makes the environment unfavourable for disease causing organisms.

Living Things and Nature

According to Native Americans who have great respect for herbs, all natural things have to exist harmoniously for people to enjoy good health. This harmony includes plants, animals and human beings. Such harmony ensures the society is not only healthy physically, but also emotionally and spiritually.

In fact, it is in this spirit of harmony that Native Americans would come together when one among them was suffering – during ill health – to conduct healing ceremonies. During such times, they would pray and dance to special songs, and sometimes chant select kinds of mantras as they administered herbal treatments. Obviously, herbal-based treatments are not something new.

Native Americans Approach to Medicine

Native Americans discovered the healthy potency of herbs a long time ago. They realized there were leaves, roots and other parts of plants they could use to treat certain ailments prevalent in their communities.

There are many tribes considered to be native to North America. In fact, there are said to be in excess of 2,000, and every one of them had its rituals and ceremonies that were carried out at different times. Different tribes sometimes carried out various healing processes differently; and when such knowledge and accompanying processes are consolidated, they form a rich bank of knowledge and skills important in natural treatments.

They had healers or medicine men and women, whom the foreigners who settled in the country commonly referred to as 'Shamans.' These traditional healers not only played the role of physicians, but one of priests as well. They would be the link between the earthly happenings and the spiritual world. This was very important in the welfare of the community because Native Americans believed disease was not only a natural malaise, but also a supernatural one.

These traditional healers wore masks for easy identification, and for the purpose of scaring away evil spirits those masks were purposely given a grotesque look. These spirits were targeted because they were said to be the cause of diseases and other forms of pain.

As the healers performed the rituals to exorcise demons, they would dance around the afflicted person as they shook rattles and beat drums. This was the supernatural aspect of the traditional treatment. For the natural aspect, the healers would use natural products derived from animals and plants in various healing procedures.

Some of the procedures these healers used alongside herbal treatments had a bit of sophistication too – like those involving the use of suction tubes, or just cups, to purify and purge bodily substances.

Qualifications of a Traditional Healer

Those who qualified to practice as traditional healers often came from a family with a history of traditional healing; many generations before them practiced traditional medicine.

Others were just interested in learning the art of traditional healing, having been inspired by their own experiences. The common denominator between these two categories of traditional healers was that they would both begin practising under the supervision of an established traditional healer; a form of apprenticeship that took a reasonable period of time.

Tools Used by Traditional Healers

Native American healers used natural tools in their treatment procedures. These included feathers, animal skins and shells, bones, crystals, and such other materials.

As for the feathers, they were instrumental in transmitting messages from the natural world to that of the supernatural; messages that traversed the air and the wind. Sometimes the traditional healer would enter into a trance, and it is in this state where he would receive guiding messages from the spirits.

The healers would have traditional medications tied into bundles and wrapped in cloth, and they would carry them carefully in their hands as they performed the rituals. The medications contained in every bundle depended on the issue at hand. For example, bundles meant to be used during festivals would have different content from those meant to be used in healing some type of disease.

Native Americans would also sometimes make use of medicine pipes; items that reflected the manner in which life flows. There are times when the healers used the pipes alongside bundles of medicine. It was believed that as the healers smoked from the pipes, the smoke they emitted carried prayers for direct delivery to the spirits.

Role of Herbs in Healing

It is worth noting that conventionally people thought of herbs as plants that are not woody. However, the term 'herb' is today commonly used in reference to any of the several plant parts, like the leaves, roots, bark and others, from which one can extract medicinal substances. Non-woody plants are, nevertheless, are still referred to as herbs; but the term is not exclusive to them.

Many of the herbs used for their medicinal value are also valuable as food, while others are valued for their flavor or fragrance. This means not only are herbs great sources of medicine; they are also rich sources of natural spices and perfume. Also, just as in ancient days, some herbs are used in rituals of a spiritual nature.

Indians are among the world's civilizations of old most famous for their practice in traditional medicine. Over the years, they have continued to source herbal extracts from their forests; and even today they harvest plant parts from there to extract herbal medicine. It is said the number of herbal treatments Indians have found in forests are in excess of 8,000.

It is not surprising that the Native Americans, who are actually Americans of Indian descent, continued to practice herbal medicine in North America. These natives comprised different tribes, which include the Cherokee, the Cheyenne, the Apache, the Crow people, and others.

According to the World Health Organization or WHO, 80% of the world's population benefit primarily from use of herbal remedies. The organization also indicates that there are 21,000 species of plants with potential to be used as herbal treatments.

One of the reasons herbal treatments have become very popular is they are believed to be safe. For those thought to have side-effects, they have been found to be minimal. Another reason is both men and women, can benefit from herbal remedies.

Another great reason herbal medication continues to be popular is some of them have capacity to treat maladies modern medicine cannot heal. It is also beneficial that some herbs have the capacity to treat ailments common in communities. Such herbs include Aloe and the Tulsi or Basil, and even Ginger, Neem and Turmeric; herbs which are very common in day-to-day use.

CHAPTER 2

MOST VALUABLE US HERBS

There are thousands of herbs available for use in North America. Among them is Abies Balsamea, Agave, Agrimony, Aloe Vera, Amaranth, Angelica, Echinacea, Mint and many others.

Herbs Available in North America

Other herbs one can find in North America include Alder, Arsemart and Indian Ginseng; Balsam fir and Balsam root, the Beech and Barberry, Bearberry and Black cohosh, Chamomile, Cranberry, Dandelion, Echinacea, Feverfew, Geranium, Hawthorn, Hyssop, Juniper, Lemon Balm, Maple, Nettle, Oregon Grape, Passionflower, Prickly Pear, Redroot, Slippery Elm, Toothwort, Usnea, Violet, Water Birch, Yarrow and Zizia Aurea.

Popular Medicinal Herbs, Where to Find Them, How to Identify Them & What they Treat

Abies Balsamea

Abies Balsamea is found within the forests in the northern parts of the US, and also the southern areas of Canada.

The Abies Balsamea is actually the tree known as the Balsam Fir, which is perennially green. It grows very tall and can even attain the height of 65ft. The tree has a grey bark that often discharges sap. It also has capacity to alter its look in its different stages of development. Hence the barks of young Abies Balsamea trees are smooth while those of the old ones are coarse.

This tree has leaves whose top section is needle-like and green, while their bottom part is white. It also has long red or purplish cones that measure around 4 inches.

Extract from the bark of Abies Balsamea is medicinal. It is great at reducing fever and detoxifying the body by stimulating the body to sweat. Also, herbal tea made from this plant has been known to treat issues of respiration. This is because of its astringent properties.

Sap can also be extracted from the herb for treatment of burns and cuts. People also lick this sap for the sake of preventing colds or sore throat.

Agave

Agave can be found in Nevada and other states in the southern parts of the US like California and Arizona; and also within Mexico.

The agave is a perennial herb whose leaves have a greenish, and sometimes greyish, color. It develops from a short stem in the middle from where the succulent, long and pointed leaves emerge. Due to the prominence and layout of the leaves, it is not easy to see the stem at a glance. This plant is known to produce one flower at a time, which emerges from the spike at the center of the plant. This flower ends up dying after a relatively short time.

Agave produces sap and juices that experts often use in the process of tequila making. Others use it to make progesterone, which is often prescribed to pregnant women.

The sap from this herb is also great at mending wounds as an emergency measure.

Agrimony

Agrimony thrives well in all parts of the US, but it is mostly found in meadows and along the margins of woody areas.

Agrimony, a perennial herb, emerges from a tiny rhizome. It has an upright stem that can reach the height of 30 inches. The leaves of agrimony are narrow and their margins are serrated; and every one of those leaves is accompanied by an additional pair of leaves that are smaller in size. These two other leaves have a somewhat different shape from the main ones.

The flowers of this herb are yellow in color, and they develop in cluster form at the top edge of the herb. Every one of those flowers has 5 petals and stamens that protrude out of it.

For use in modern medicine, some extract is derived from the agrimony leaves and processed to produce astringents and diaphoretics. It is also used as febrifuge. However, for traditional use, a decoction can be prepared from the agrimony root for treatment of diarrhea and fever. There is also a way tea is prepared from the plant leaves and the flowers for the sake of treating UTIs or Urinary Tract Infections.

Alder

Alder can be found in all wet areas of Canada and the US.

The Alder is actually a tree whose height can reach 70ft. It has a bark that covers its entire large trunk. The trunk of a young alder tree is smooth with a greyish color, while its older version is coarse and has a whitish color.

This medicinal tree has oval shaped leaves whose tips are pointed. Also, its leaves are serrated. The tree's male flowers are long and have a greenish-yellowish color, while the females are tiny and reddish. While the male flowers protrude facing downward, the female develop into cones that later produce seeds with a flat shape.

The bark of the alder is used for medicinal purposes in modern day practice. The solution produced using water is used as an astringent or tonic. It also has a cathartic effect.

Nevertheless, traditionally a concoction was prepared from the female flowers and used for treatment of Sexually Transmitted Diseases or STDs, such as gonorrhoea. The male flower, on its part, has been made into a poultice that was consumed for purposes of stimulating bowel movement whenever a person had constipation. The flower poultices were also used to treat infections in wounds as well as on the skin.

Another medicinal use for this herb came from its leaves, which when dried were used to make tea with anti-inflammatory properties. If someone's skin had a rash, the herbal tea would be used to wash the affected part and it would heal.

The most popular use today is in the treatment of sore throat. People gurgle decoctions produced by boiling the inner part of the bark, which is normally made from fresh bark. All the bark actually has the effect of an astringent or a febrifuge.

Aloe Vera

Although aloe Vera can be found in the southern areas of the US, it is most prevalent in southeastern parts of the country.

The aloe Vera has leaves of olive-green in colour, but sometimes they are yellowish. Right from the plant's base, the long leaves form a rosette as they develop to become pointed and tooth-edged. This plant has leaves that are succulent and pointed; and it produces flowers that emerge in tubular form in groups of red or even yellow. These flowers form a spike in the middle of the plant as they develop.

When the leaves of the Aloe Vera are still fresh, they are used in the treatment of wounds and insect bites, as well as burns. There is also an ancient use that many people do not know about, and this is the drying of these leaves and then grinding them to convert them into powder form. This is used for inhibiting bleeding in an open wound. This powder is also effective in the treatment of blisters because it absorbs moisture and prevents infection.

The same powder can be diluted using water, and then drank to help get rid of intestinal worms.

Angelica

Angelica thrives well in the moist lowlands of North America, mostly in the states of the North-east.

The stems of the angelica plant are thick and purple, and their height can go up to 6ft. The plant has huge leaves, with smaller ones shaped in oval and grouped in threes of fives. The flowers are white, small, and grouped to form umbels.

The angelica is very much like the hemlock, but for safety reasons, there is need for proper identification. While a broken hemlock stem or leaf emits the smell of urine, those of angelica have a smell similar to that of celery.

A poultice made from a fresh angelica root can be rubbed onto a swollen joint to fight inflammation and relieve pain. This root poultice is also effective when used in any other part of the body where the tissue has been injured. Whether the swelling is mild or severe, this herbal treatment is effective in reducing inflammation and easing pain.

Arsemart

Arsemart can be found anywhere in the US, as long as the area is wet.

Other names arsemart goes by are Water Pepper and Marsh Pepper Smartweed. This herb has an annual lifespan and grows to a height of 30 inches.

It has a taproot that penetrates the earth to a depth of around 3ft, and so it is not easy to kill it. The stem of the herb is straight with a greenish-red colour, while its narrow leaves are hairy. The flowers this plant produces are pink in colour.

The poultice and the juice from any of the arsemart's parts can be used in treating ulcers. Either of the two can also be used in the treatment of a swollen joint. The herbal extracts from this plant can be used both externally and internally; meaning they can be consumed or applied on the skin or the surface of the affected part of the body.

This herb is also effective in the treatment of toothaches. Tea can also be made from the leaves or flowers of this plant and drank for the sake of eliminating parasitic worms in the intestines.

Barberry

The forests of Canada and the northern parts of the US make great habitats for the herb, Barberry.

The barberry is a shrub with thorny branches, whose height can reach 8ft. It has succulent leaves that appear to have teeth on the edges; and these emerge in clusters.

The barberry flowers, which are yellow in colour, appear close to the branch tips. There are 6 sepals per flower, and as they develop they turn scarlet.

The leaves, berries and bark of the barberry all have medicinal value, and when a decoction or other mixture is being prepared, either water or alcohol can be used. These parts have antiseptic and carminative properties, and they are also great for febrifuge.

For this reason, decoctions from this herb have been used for years for treatment of diarrhoea. Its preparations are also used to treat sore throat by gargling; and mouth sores and wounds through direct application.

Leaf decoctions can also be used in detoxifying the liver, while a poultice from the roots in their raw or cooked form can be used to enhance salivation and subsequently stimulation of the appetite for invalids.

Bearberry

Bearberry thrives in the forests of Canada, and those within the northern and western parts of the US.

The bearberry is a very short shrub that remains green all year round. Its leaves are smooth and also thick. This plant begins flowering in spring and produces tiny flowers that are pinkish-white in colour. These flowers that appear in clusters emerge towards the topmost part of the stem.

The bearberry has round fruits that are red in colour, each of which has around three seeds in it. The seeds of the bearberry are pretty hard.

For the bearberry, it is the leaves that are medicinal. Their extracts can be dissolved in water or alcohol and then consumed for their diuretic and astringent properties. A poultice made from the leaves is often applied onto wounds to inhibit bleeding, while decoctions are prepared from the leaves or even the berries for treatment of kidney or bladder related issues. These decoctions also have analgesic properties, albeit mild.

Traditionally, salve extracted from the leaves of this herb would be applied on rashes or even sores, after beeswax had been added to it to make it reasonably thick.

Beech

Beech is found in the eastern parts of the US and also in the southern areas of Canada.

The beech is a large tree that does best in sandy soils or those that are chalky. It can grow up to 140ft high and its trunk can expand up to a thickness of 21ft. The beech also has brittle wood that is strong and durable.

The bark of the beech tree has antacid and antipyretic properties. Other medicinal properties this bark possesses include anti-tussive, meaning it can suppress coughs; as well as being a great expectorant. It also has odontalgic properties, which means it has the capacity to suppress toothaches.

Beech tree branches also have antiseptic properties, and so a form of tar is made by boiling them and distilling the solution that can be consumed. This solution is also stimulating and thus enhances the process of expectoration, and when used externally it is great at treating skin ailments.

Black Cohosh

Black cohosh can be found in some areas of Canada, and also in various parts of the US like Maine, Ontario, the western part of Missouri as well as Indiana, the southern parts of Georgia, and the western areas of North Carolina.

The black cohosh is a perennial herb that grows in the woodlands, and it is one of the buttercup species. It has tiny plumes that comprise tiny flowers, which are white and shaped in form of a star. These flowery plumes can grow up to a height of 8ft; although often they only get up to around 5ft.

Extracts from black cohosh are used to make oral solutions that have been found to reduce menopause symptoms. The medicinal parts of this herb include its roots and the rhizome after it has been dried.

Black Gum

Black gum is often referred to as black tupelo, sour gum or simply tupelo; and it is growing naturally in the north-eastern parts of the US, southern areas of Ontario, within the southern and central parts of Florida, and the east area of Texas.

The black gum is also referred to as black tupelo, and its scientific name is Nyssa sylvatica. It is a tree of the deciduous type that grows up to medium size, although at times it can become large.

In the month of September, the leaves of the black gum tree are green, but in due course they become intensely red with some orange hues and others that are yellow and even purple. Because of this unique combination of colours, the black gum is often sought to use in landscaping of homes.

Liquid from black gum roots is used to treat eye ailments, while infusions made out of bark extracts are used for gynaecological purposes on a woman in labour. It has also been found that decoctions made out of the plant bark are good for treating pulmonary tuberculosis when used in a bath.

Black Haw

The shrub that is black haw grows naturally in the central and the southern woodlands of North America.

The black haw, which is a close relative of the honeysuckle, has a bark that is reddish, which is used in preparation of herbal teas or even tinctures. Most users of the herb prefer harvesting the bark during fall. Flowers that are white in colour emerge in clusters during spring, and subsequently haws, which can be described as drupes develop during autumn. These haws have a yellowish-green colour and look like berries.

Natural extracts from the black haw are diuretics, meaning they have the capacity to increase urine with the effect of relieving the body of excess fluid; in short avoiding unwanted retention of fluid.

The roots of the plant are the main parts used for production of herbal medicine, which is also used during menstruation and childbirth. The medications from these roots help to alleviate pain and also relax the uterine muscles; hence cramps are reduced during menstruation and spasms minimized during childbirth. This means not only does the treatment bring comfort to the individuals concerned, but the risk of miscarriage is also minimized.

Bloodroot

The bloodroot, which is also known as sanguinaria canadensis, can be found in the eastern parts of North America and also Canada.

The bloodroot is an herb whose flowers comprise 8 petals each. These flowers are white and shaped like a cup. Their stamens, which are bright yellow, emerge from the middle of the flower, which develops to a length of between 4cm – 6cm. The stalk that holds the flower is reddish and has a length of around 20cm.

The seeds of the bloodroot have elaisosomes, structures that are abundantly fleshy for the purpose of attracting ants. These ants act as the medium for dispersing the herb's seeds.

Extracts from the bloodroot plant are used to treat vomiting and to reduce toothaches. They are also used where people have problems emptying their bowels. Ordinarily it is the plant rhizome, the stem-like part that develops underground that is used for production of herbal medicine.

The bloodroot has also been found to help in cases of laryngitis or where a person's throat goes hoarse, as well as sore throat that is clinically termed as pharyngitis. It also helps to treat nasal polyps and warts, even as it reduces joint pain and muscle aches.

Blue False Indigo

Blue false indigo, also known as Blue Wild Indigo or Wild Blue Indigo, is also called Baptisia Australis; and it is found in the central as well as eastern areas of North America.

The false indigo perennial herb is upright and shrubby in form, and its leaves are bluish green in colour. It has colourful flowers and unique-looking pods, making the plant distinctly showy. This herb belongs is one of the pea species, and like the rest it fertilizes itself by fixing of nitrogen.

Decoctions are made from the false indigo roots for treatment of wounds, skin, and other external parts of the body. For example, a decoction can be made to treat an ear infection or even to treat a nasal infection. It can also be used to treat ulcers of the mouth, tonsillitis, and throat issues. False indigo extracts are effective because of the plant's antiseptic properties.

Decoctions from this plant's roots have also been found to be helpful in treating Leukorrhea, which is a condition where a woman releases discharges of a white, yellow or even green coloured discharge from her vagina. Sometimes such discharge occurs normally, but if it is a result of infection, douching with the decoction can be helpful as far as treatment is concerned. In general, false indigo decoctions are good at stimulating the body's immune response.

Boneset

The boneset is naturally found in North America's wetlands, particularly the eastern areas of Canada and the US. The herb is found in states like Florida, Louisiana, Nebraska, Texas and such others. In Canada, boneset grows along the shores.

The boneset is a perennial herb that grows to a height of between 0.6 and 1.8 meters. It is a perennial plant that is not only coarse but also rough and hairy, and it is mostly found in wet areas. Its leaves are wrinkled and toothed, and with a lance shape. They come together at the base as they surround the stem of the plant.

The boneset produces disk-like flowers that are small and white in colour, and which have many heads. These heads ultimately form a flat cluster.

Extracts from the boneset herb are good at reducing fever and alleviating constipation. They are also used to enhance release of urine. Other ailments said to be treated using boneset include influenza, rheumatism, inflammation of the nose, swine flu and pneumonia. The herb is also credited with treatment of dengue fever, acute bronchitis and excess retention of fluids.

These extracts are also known for their stimulant properties, and their capacity to facilitate sweating. The medicinal material of the plant is normally extracted from the flowers and the leaves, in their dried form.

Buckthorn (Cascara Sagrada)

The buckthorn naturally grows in the western areas of North America, and in Canada there are people who plant it.

The buckthorn, also called Cascara Sagrada, is a tall shrub that can grow to a height of 20ft. It has a loosely formed crown that spreads out of several stems that emerge from the ground.

This plant looks like a small tree and has silvery projections that look like corks. It is important that people be cautious when harvesting parts of this plant because its bark, which is brown in colour, also resembles that of a native plum.

Buckhorn bark is used in detoxifying the body the natural way. It also provides the extracts to treat constipation as well as other varying digestion related problems. This is because it has a substance known as anthraquinones that possesses laxative capability. Primarily, the compounds in this herb help to form stool into larger pieces that are also softer, making the movement of bowels relatively easy.

California Poppy

The California poppy naturally grows along the North American slopes; in the western parts of Oregon, Baja California, and elsewhere.

The leaves of a California poppy are one or two inches in length, and in their segmented form they form a rosette right at the base of the herb. When the few flowers appear, they have four petals that are 2.5inch in length.

The parts of the California poppy that emerge above ground level are used to produce medicine, which treats different ailments among them insomnia or other sleep issues. Among the medical conditions treated using this herb includes one related with the liver and another to the bladder. Consequently, it is found to be effective in stopping children's habit of bedwetting.

Catnip

Catnip, an herb that shares the same family as mint, can be found within North American, although it is native to Europe as well as Asia.

The catnip is greenish-grey in colour, and it grows up to a height of around 3ft. The leaves of this herb are jagged and shaped like a heart, while its stem is thick and hairy.

The flowers of this herb form big clusters when they bloom, and these clusters are at the plant top looking like tiny tubular openings.

The flowers of the catnip as well as its leaves have medicinal value, and they are normally used to prepare tea with calming properties. The decoction from this herb has been credited with treating indigestion and cramping of the intestines, as well as raising a person's appetite level.

Cattail

The cattail grows in the Canadian waterways and within the marshes. This herb, which originated in Europe, can now be found in the US and also Canada.

Cattails are plants that can grow to a height of 8ft, with the length of their leaves being between 5 and 9 feet. These plants have strong stalks whose leaves are pointed, and the plants thrive in shallow waters or in damp soils. Cattail herbs form spikes that are brown in colour, and which exist in thick colonies. The flowers of this plant emerge out of the spikes.

The root of the cattail can be ground and the powder used as poultice to treat burns as well as sores, and even cuts and stings. Flower fuzz can also be used for treatment of burns as well as sores; and for children it is good at preventing chafing.

Chamomile

The chamomile, also known as Matricaria recutita, can be found in North America, although its continents of origin were Europe, Asia and also Africa.

Chamomile, an annual herb, produces flowers that look like daisies; whose petals are white. These petals circle a yellowish middle part that has the shape of a cone. The flowers of this edible plant do not grow beyond a length of $2^1/_2$ cm.

The inside disk of the chamomile florets that happen to be yellow in colour, have great healing properties.

The preparations made from this herb are great at treating inflammations and hay fever, as well as problems related to menstruation. They also treat muscle spasms and gastro-intestinal conditions.

Cicely

The herb, cicely, can be found in many locations of North America, but its place of origin was Europe.

The cicely herb has a hollow and round stem that is also hairy. Those stem hairs have a soft feel. The cicely plant has leaves with random marks that are chalky in look, and seeds close to those of cucumbers. As the seeds develop, they become edible as they acquire a blackish look.

Every part of the cicely plant inclusive of the seeds has healing properties. These parts can be prepared to serve as expectorants, where they are effective in alleviating coughs. They also serve as treatments for stomach problems, as they treat flatulence and act as gentle stomach stimulants.

Over the years, the decoction from the cicely plant root has been found to be an effective antiseptic that treats snake bites as well as dog bites.

Cow Parsnip

The cow parsnip can be found in the grasslands of the US, as well as in the meadows and Riparian areas.

The cow parsnip has big leaves each of which is dissected to form three leaflets. A leaflet of this plant has lobes that are rounded in shape, and these lobes are pointed.

Every part of the cow parsnip can be used for treatment purposes, as they have antispasmodic and carminative properties, as well as a stimulating effect. They also have capacity to fight rheumatism.

The leaves of this herb are used to make tonic drinks with the capacity to treat colds and sooth a sore throat.

Some people also make infusions of young leaves when they are still fresh, and use them to treat diarrhea. Also, these infusions are effective in eliminating warts.

As for the plant's roots, they are used to make tea, which, when drank helps to treat indigestion and stomach cramps, as well as colds and rheumatism and related ailments.

Damiana

This herb known as damiana or passifloraceae can be found in Texas and the West Indies, but mostly within the regions of Central America.

Damian is an herb that grows up to around 60 centimeters in height. Its leaves are a pale green, and they develop to yellowish brown in dried form. These leaves, whose edges are jagged, are significantly narrow, and they often grow to between 15 to 25 millimeters.

Leaves of the Damian herb are dried and used in preparation of an herbal tea that treats headaches. It is also used to treat a nervous stomach, and to boost and maintain mental health as well as deliver physical endurance.

The tea made from this plant has also been found to help solve issues of a sexual nature, serving as a form of aphrodisiac.

American Cranberry

The American cranberry is native to the northern areas of the US, where it was mostly consumed by the native tribes.

The American cranberry is a deciduous plant whose height can reach 15ft. Its leaves resemble those of maple; and they are lobed and are dark-green in colour. Over time, this greenish colour develops a red or yellow shade, and can even turn purple as autumn sets in.

The flowers of the American cranberry are white in colour, and they develop into numerous red fruits that are a favourite for birds.

Although traditionally cranberries were used in the treatment of arrow wounds, today they are mostly used to fight infections of the bladder.

Dandelion

The dandelion has a natural habitat in North America, although some of its species originated in Europe.

The easiest way to identify a dandelion is through its basal leaves that emerge from the stem's base, and also through the yellow flowers they produce.

There are other plants that look like the dandelion, but the dandelion stands out owing to its hairless leaves. The edges of dandelion leaves are toothed, while the stems of its flowers are hollow. The major parts of a dandelion – the root, the stem and the leaves – produce a whitish milky sap.

While the dandelion leaves have capacity to act as a mild laxative and hence enhance digestion, the plant's roots have properties that help in solving problems of the liver and the kidneys, as well as the gallbladder. To a certain extent, the plant can reduce diabetic problems.

The roots are effective as treatments because of their detoxification capacity; and the plant in general helps to boost the body's immunity.

Devil's Club

The devil's club is found along the coast of Alaska and in areas to the south of that state, where the forests are properly drained. It is also found to the east of California and the Rocky Mountains. There is also a portion to the north of Lake Superior where the herb grows naturally.

The devil's club is a deciduous plant that often grows to between one to three meters in height. It has extraordinarily large leaves and thin spines that are very sharp, and which cover not only the stem but also the leaves. This feature makes the plant stand out among other plants.

The length of the spines is normally between 5 and 10 millimeters and the color of the stem is a light tan. Also, the stem looks crooked.

The herb's root has a bark whose inside part is credited with having medicinal properties. The plant stem is also known for its effective in treatment of various ailments.

In particular, extracts from the plant's bark are used to boost appetite and to purify blood. They are also used in easy expulsion of afterbirth, so that the menstrual flow that occurs soon after can be well regulated.

Root infusions are used externally for treatment of diphtheria.

Douglas Maple

Douglas maple grows naturally on the south-eastern region of Alaska and the British Columbia, as well as the south-western parts of Alberta. The herb can also be found in the states of California as well as New Mexico, and to the south of Oregon. Other areas of the US where the herb grows include eastern Idaho and also Montana.

The Douglas maple is a shrub that has a crown and several stems that grow upwards. The plant is tall and its crown is narrow; and the color of the plant's bark when mature is grey in color, but it is red when very young.

The Douglas maple plant is effective in treatment of nausea. Substances for treatment are extracted from the plant's bark and its wood, and often from the twigs as well.

The concoction made can be used in enhancing lactation, and also to treat nausea and diarrhea.

Echinacea

Echinacea, also known as purple coneflower, can be found within the prairies and meadows of the US, and where the prairies are moist. This means one can find Echinacea in the states of Ohio, Michigan, Iowa, Georgia and also Louisiana.

The Echinacea has narrow leaves that are tooth-edged, and they are lance-shaped. Their upper area is usually a dark-greenish colour, and it has some sparsely distributed whitish hairs.

The flowers of Echinacea have petals that form the shape of a cone, and they have a purple-magenta colour.

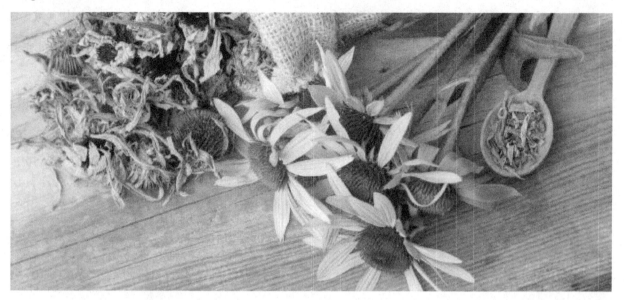

The root of the Echinacea plant as well as the aerial sections of the plant has medicinal properties; the latter parts being used to make herbal tea. The extracts from this plant are used in treating common colds and coughs, infections of the respiratory system, bronchitis, and other inflammations.

Feverfew

The feverfew herb, which originated in Europe, can now be found in North America. The species known as Wild Feverfew can be found within New England in the US.

The feverfew herbs usually form a form of bush as they grow, and their height can go up to around 50cm. This plant has tiny flowers that are white in colour, and whose middle area is yellow. The scent the leaves of these plants emit is sometimes like citrus.

Feverfew has leaves which, when dried, produce material of great medicinal value. Nevertheless, every one of the plant's parts that develop above the surface of the earth has medicinal properties.

The extracts from this plant are effective at treating fevers and migraines, as well as rheumatoid arthritis, aches of the stomach and the teeth, arthritis and insect bites.

Frasera

The herb known as frasera also goes by the name the yellow gentian, and also the American columbo. It can be found within the southern parts of Ontario in Canada, and also on the eastern areas of the US. It is also present on the south-eastern parts of the US.

The frasera herb produces flowers with 4 petals; and these flowers are hermaphroditic as far as reproduction is concerned. The petals have purple dots that draw pollinators close, and these dots are often referred to as nectar guides.

The frasera plant as a whole is of medicinal value. The leaves and the roots can be dried and powdered, and in that state the plant is used to treat several ailments such as colds and asthma. The plant is also be used to alleviate issues of digestion, including diarrhea.

Gentian

The gentian herb, which is also referred to as the bottle gentian, is found within the north-eastern parts of the US. It particularly thrives where the soils are rich and moist.

The gentian herb is alternately called the Gentiana. It produces narrow leaves that are green in colour, and flowers whose petals are sometimes 4 and other times 5 in number.

These petals normally form the shape of a bell or trumpet, and though they are ordinarily blue in colour, they sometimes come in other colors like white or yellow, American Elderberry

The roots of the gentian plant have medicinal properties. They have bitter substances that help to treat problems of digestion. As they treat bloating, heartburn and diarrhea, they also enhance appetite. Sometimes the plant's bark is also used for medicinal purposes, treating not only fever but also muscle spasms.

Geranium

The geranium herb is found in very many species, and some of them grow in North America and also Hawaii. Within the US, this herb can be found in the states of North Dakota, South Dakota, Louisiana and Oklahoma; while within Canada the geranium grows in Ontario as well as Quebec.

The geranium plant produces leaves that produce a distinctive scent, often an aromatic one, after being rubbed or just pressed. These leaves are fleshy and round in shape, and sometimes they are shaped like a hand.

The plant itself, though herbaceous, sometimes develops like a woody plant. Its flowers develop in clusters, and their colors can vary from white to violet or red or even pinkish.

A poultice made out of geranium's ground roots is effective in the treatment of burns, and it is also used in the treatment of haemorrhoids. Traditionally, people would grind the roots and the leaves of this herb, and the poultice produced would be used in treating not only sore throats, but also serious ailments such as diarrhea, cholera and gonorrhoea.

Modern day users have found that oil can be produced from geraniums and used in treating infections and inflammations, while also acting as an anti-oxidant.

Ginseng

The ginseng herb, which is also known as Panax quinquefolius, is found in North America, in areas like around the Great Lakes and the Gulf of Mexico. In Canada, the herb has always thrived in Quebec as well as Manitoba.

The ginseng is a perennial plant with leaves that develop at a stem's end. Every one of these leaves has between 3 and 5 leaflets; the reason the ginseng leaves are said to be compound.

When mature, the herb has between 6 and 20 flowers in cluster form, whose colour is a white-green. In due course, these flowers produce berries that are red in colour.

The ginseng has a fleshy root that looks like the leg of a human being, though dependent on how old the herb is the root can look a human being in shape. The shape of the ginseng root actually changes to become forked as it crosses the 3rd year mark in age. The ginseng root is ready for harvesting after it has attained the age of between 5 and 7 years, by which stage it might be as long as 12 inches in length.

The roots of the ginseng plant – the main one as well as the lateral ones – are used alongside their hairs to produce material potent with healing properties. The plant extract is used to treat inflammations, to regulate the level of glucose in the blood, boost a person's immunity, improve the function of the brain, and to reduce fatigue.

This plant has also been found to have anti-oxidant properties, as well as the capacity to reduce symptoms associated with erectile dysfunction.

Goldenrod

The goldenrod herb is a perennial herb found in North America and even Hawaii; and many other parts of the world. There are over a hundred species of goldenrod all over the world, and it has been noted that almost every state in the US has one or more species of this medicinal herb.

The goldenrod has leaves that are a bit jagged along their edges, but which are otherwise smooth. The stems of the plant are strong, and the way to distinguish them from other similar plants known for their toxicity is the way those of goldenrod develop. They are not known for branching out like those look-alikes.

Usually the flowers of the goldenrod are yellow in colour, but there is the white goldenrod whose flowers are a different colour. These flowers sometimes form a narrow pyramid as they grow, which can attain a height of up to between 2 and 16 inches.

The sections of the goldenrod plant that develop above the ground surface have medicinal properties; the most potent being the flowers and the leaves of the plant.

This is a plant known for treating very serious ailments like diabetes, arthritis and asthma; but it is also credited with capacity to treat gout, liver enlargement, tuberculosis, hemorrhoids, and internal bleeding in general.

Traditional native Americans would use the plant extract rinse the mouth in a bid to cure mouth and throat inflammations. They would also use it not only to fight pain and reduce swellings, but also as diuretics that would enhance the flow of urine. They also credited the plant with helping in stopping muscle spasms.

Goldenseal

The goldenseal grows within the Blue Ridge mountains of the US, and other areas of North America.

The goldenseal is a plant whose leaves are a shiny green, and which resemble maples. This plant produces only one flower that is white in colour, and whose stamens are yellow. The sepals of the flower drop as the flower opens, and after that fruits are produced that are red in colour. These fruits are actually tiny berries, and they form a cluster.

The root of the goldenseal plant is rich in healing properties, and it is normally dried for use. The product is then used externally on the skin for treatment of rashes and itching; and it is also effective in the treatment of eczema, blisters, and acne. Other ailments effectively treated using extracts from goldenseal include ringworms, herpes, cold sores, and even dandruff.

Goldenseal is also sought after when people want to make mouthwash for treatment of sore gums and other infections of the mouth.

Extracts from this plant have also been credited in producing an eyewash that treats inflammations of the eyes, and very importantly, the eye infection often referred to as 'pink eye.'

Gooseberry

There are many species of the gooseberry herb. Some of them are found in the north-eastern parts of the US and the northern and central parts of the US. The gooseberry herb is also found in US parts next to Canada.

The gooseberry plant has leaves that are dark green in colour, and which produce flowers shaped like a bell. These flowers produce berries that are greenish yellow in colour, although sometimes they turn red. The berries, which are often a single inch in length, have numerous tiny seeds. The gooseberry plants usually develop into a tiny bush.

The entire gooseberry plant has medicinal properties. This means medicinal extracts can be made from the fruits, seeds, or even the leaves. Because the plant was very much valued by the Native Americans as a source of medicine, it is often referred to as the Indian gooseberry.

The plant is great at lowering the level of cholesterol in the body, and also in reducing incidents of heartburn. As far as reduction of cholesterol is concerned, the medicinal properties of this plant target the fats within the blood, hence treating the condition of dyslipidemia. The condition of dyslipidemia simply means there are excess lipids in the blood, where lipids refer to cholesterol and triglycerides.

Gravel Root

The gravel root, which is also known as eupatorium purpureum, is a perennial herb commonly referred to as 'queen of the meadow. It can be found in the eastern region of North America. This herb thrives in swampy meadows.

The herb is especially present in Florida in the US, and in the southern regions of Canada.

The gravel root is an herb that also goes by the name kidney root, trumpet weed or eupatorium purpureum, among others. It has leaves whose under-parts have tiny bristles. Its root develops in bulb form that is just as edible as the parts that grow above the Earth's surface.

The medicinal portions of the plant include the bulb and the root, and the sections over ground level in general. Though used sparingly, the extracts from this plant are effective in treating UTI or urinary tract infections, and other ailments associated with the urinary tract.

The plant is also credited with the treatment of kidney stones, bladder infections, pain during urination, and other health conditions affecting the urethra and the prostate.

Gutierrezia

Gutierrezia is an herb that grows in the western parts of the US and parts of Canada. The northern parts of Mexico particularly have this herb, and the eastern areas of Minnesota also have it. Generally the herb is found in several parts of North America and is largely considered to be a weed.

The Gutierrezia is among the medicinal flowering plants available in North America. Its scientific name is Gutierrezia sarothrae, but it also goes by the names snakeweed, matchweed or broomweed.

Sometimes people confuse Gutierrezia with the rabbitbrush; but the easiest way to distinguish the two is to notice that Gutierrezia has gray flowers that are not present in rabbitbrush.

Gutierrezia is medicinal overall; meaning that every part of the plant has some medicinal value. The leaves are the most popular as far as treatment is concerned, as they are used to make infusions that treat coughs, fevers and colds in general.

In fact, as far as treatment of fever is concerned, the plant extracts are used in bath form. This bath is also effective in treating sores within the respiratory system. It is also credited in treating sores of a venereal nature.

Fresh leaves have also been used to produce a poultice, and in its moist form the poultice effectively heals bruises and wounds as well as sprains. It is also used in the treatment of insect bites and to stop nosebleeds.

Hawthorn

The hawthorn plant is a shrub that is found in temperate areas, including those of North America.

The hawthorn plant is thorny and it produces flowers with 5 petals. These flowers can have different colors; white, pink or even red. The plant produces fruits that are drupe-like; having one seed and being fleshy. These fruits are red in colour, and people call them berries when they find them being sold.

The medicinal parts of the hawthorn plants include the plant berries, flowers and the leaves. They produce extracts used in the treatment of heart diseases like chest pains, irregular heartbeat and CHF or Congestive Heart Failure.

The plant is particularly credited with regulating blood pressure; treating blood pressure whether it is too high or too low. It is also liked for its capacity to manage the condition of the arteries, so that the arteries do not harden too much; in short treating the condition known as atherosclerosis. The hawthorn plant is also effective in mitigating high cholesterol.

Healall

Healall also goes by the names selfheal and even Lanceleaf selfheal. It can be found in North America; usually along the sides of the road and within clear meadows.

The Healall herb has the tendency to bend when it attains a particular height, and gradually its tip touches the ground and develops fresh roots.

The healall plant is used in treatment when its leaves are dried and made into a solution. This medicinal solution has been found effective in the treatment of bacterial infections, and also inflammations.

It is also used for soothing burns, clearing acne and enhancing healing of injuries; and other times in alleviating muscle spasms.

Honeysuckle

The honeysuckle is a medicinal plant that thrives in some states of the US, like Pennsylvania, Minnesota, and the high altitude areas of North Carolina.

The honeysuckle grows to a medium size shrub, but sometimes it remains small size. It is normally found in woodlands and edges of forests. It is easy to notice it dangling shaped like a bell. The leaves of this herb are green in colour, and its flowers appear in pairs; usually beginning mid-spring and continuing toward the end of spring.

The fruit this herb produces is a beautiful red that is normally noticed at the beginning of autumn.

The parts of the honeysuckle rich in healing properties include the flowers, seeds and berries, as well as the plant's leaves.

Traditionally, extracts from this plant have been used for both internal and external use. The ailments treated include fever, various inflammations and ulcers; as well as infections of the skin.

For external use, fresh leaves are normally boiled in water. This solution is even used in healing wounds.

Hops

Hops is the name of a plant that originated in areas within the northern hemisphere, but which does particularly well in the temperate zones. The plant develops very fast as the month of April comes to an end, all the way up to the start of July.

The Hops plant is actually a shrub whose height can reach between 7 and 8 meters. This means the plant can grow at a rate of 30 centimeters per day. The plant leaves cover a vast area; can even extend to twenty square meters.

The roots of this perennial plant can grow to reach 100 meters in length in just a single season.

The flowers of the hop plant are dried before they can be used to prepare the herbal medicine. The medication produced from the hop is effective in treating anxiety and excitability, and it also helps to reduce problems with sleep, otherwise termed as insomnia.

The medication also reduces restlessness, nervousness, and tension, even as it helps to treat ADHD or Attention Deficit-Hyperactivity Disorder.

Horsetail

The horsetail plant also goes by the name Scouringrush Horsetail; and its scientific name is Equisetum hyemale. In the US, this herb thrives in the state of California – in the North, South and even Central areas of the state – and mostly within the Warner Mountains as well as the regions of the White and the Inyo Mountains.

This herb can also be found growing in moist areas, and more so within streams; where the soils are sandy. The altitude of these areas is normally between sea level and 9,800 feet high.

The horsetail is that plant often termed the bottle brush, which ordinarily grows as a weed. It is closely related to the fern and does not produce flowers.

Its other names include horse willow or shave grass, and sometimes it is even called paddock pipes or scouring rush among other names.

The parts of the horsetail plant that develop above the surface of the earth have medicinal properties. Once the herbal medicine has been produced from these parts, it is used in cases of fluid retention, otherwise termed as edema, as well as problems of the kidney and the bladder. It also treats UTI or urinary tract infections, and incontinence, which is the inability to control release of urine.

Hyssop

Hyssop, whose scientific name is Hyssopus officinalis, can be found in North America. The perennial herb is also found in Canada, often growing on the side of the road when it is not being cultivated in a garden.

Hyssop, a plant that exists in several species, including the giant hyssop, hedge hyssop and water hyssop, resembles the mint species. It emits aroma that is camphor-like.

The medicinal parts of the hyssop plant are those that develop above the surface of the ground. They are used in preparing medication for problems of a digestive nature, and those that affect the intestines.

The herbal medicine from the hyssop is also used in treating the gallbladder, colic and intestinal pains; even as it is also effective in the treatment of intestinal gas and appetite deficiency.

Winterberry

The winterberry is a shrub often found in swampy areas. In North America this tiny tree can be found in the north-eastern side; starting from Newfoundland all the way southward to Florida. It is also found to the west in states like Minnesota and Missouri.

The winterberry has dark green leaves that are slightly toothed. These leaves, which are dark green in colour, are also smooth. While their upper side is somewhat glossy, their underside is somewhat fuzzy, particularly along the veins.

This plant is actually deciduous, and it can grow to a height of up to ten feet.

The winterberry produces small flowers that are white in colour, and whose number ranges between 4 and 7 in a season.

The fruits of the winterberry are either orange or red, but sometimes they are yellow; the colors appearing distinctly brilliant after the leaves have fallen during autumn.

The part of the winterberry most potent for use as a medicine is the inside part of the bark. It not only has antiseptic and astringent properties; it also serves as a tonic. This natural medication is also cathartic; meaning it helps in the discharge of unhelpful substances from the body.

If, for some reason, a person needs to vomit, the medication from the winterberry can be used as it is an emetic.

Juniper

The juniper can be found within the Great Basin and temperate areas of North America. These include the eastern side of the state of California, the north-western areas of Nevada, the eastern parts of Oregon, some sections on the eastern side of Washington, and the south-western parts of Idaho.

The juniper is an evergreen tree that produces a cone, which resembles a tiny greenish berry. This cone is the equivalent of a fruit. In time, starting the plant's second year of existence, this berry turns a bluish-black colour.

The juniper plant produces tiny flowers that bloom toward the end of spring.

The berries of the juniper plant are medicinal; and they have been used over the years as an effective diuretic, which is also effective in the treatment of arthritis and gastro-intestinal issues.

People also use medications from juniper berries to treat diabetes and auto-immune problems.

Lady's Slipper

The lady's slipper comes in a large range of species; around 50 of them. It is mostly found in the northern region of the US that have a temperate climate, and in some areas of Canada that are moist and have acidic soils; like Newfoundland and Manitoba.

The petals of the lady's slippers fold toward their inside, forming the shape of a slipper with a middle split. The plant itself does not have a stem, and it is pinkish in colour. It is known to produce two leaves that emerge from the plant base and producing just one flower. The lady's slipper normally grows to a length of 5 centimeters.

The most potent part of the lady's slipper as far as medication is concerned is its roots. The medicine made from it is used to reduce nervousness, muscle spasms and toothaches; and also to reduce anxiety and other related ailments like insomnia, headache, hysteria and depression.

Lemon Balm

The lemon balm, also called Melissa officinalis, can be found growing naturally in North America, and is also cultivated. This perennial plant actually does well in soils that are rich and properly drained, as long as the area experiences sunshine. Nevertheless, it has the capacity to survive in areas where temperatures are as low as between -20° and -30° Fahrenheit.

The lemon balm also goes by other names like the blue balm, the balm mint, the garden balm, and even sweet balm.

The height of the plant can go up to 2ft, especially if it is not controlled. The leaves of this herb are oval-shaped, and sometimes they are shaped like a heart; basically like mint leaves. Each of the leaves grows on the opposite side of another one.

These leaves have a bright green colour on their top side, but underneath they are whitish. Nevertheless, the green can become yellowish-green according to the soil on which the plant is growing and the prevailing climate.

Among the distinctive features of the lemon balm is the plant's highly wrinkled leaves. Also, the leaves emit a tart smell that is also sweet whenever they are rubbed; essentially the way lemons do.

All the parts of the lemon balm plant have medicinal properties. The medication from this plant is generally calming and effective in enhancing sleep where individuals have had problems sleeping well.

Medications from the lemon balm also serve as great tonics; effectively treating ailments of a digestive nature.

Maidenhair Fern

The maidenhair fern is a foliage herb that can be found growing in the eastern parts of North America and even in the north-western areas of the Pacific, where there are moist woodlands.

Maidenhair ferns are known to grow in clusters, where their fiddleheads, also referred to as crosiers, are closely knit. These fiddleheads emerge out of stems that grow in a creeping manner underground.

The stems of maidenhair ferns are actually rhizomes that develop beneath the surface of the ground. In due course, these stems that happen to be black in colour begin to uncoil; and as they do so they reveal very thin branches clearly spread. These branches, alternately termed 'rachises,' bear grouped leaves; the number of these groups ranging from 5 to 7.

The fronds of the maidenhair fern, which are leafy, have great medicinal properties whether they are dried or used fresh.

The medication made from these fronds is known to fight dandruff, even as it serves as an anti-tussive and demulcent. It is also an astringent, emollient and laxative, and serves as an effective tonic and emetic.

Sugar Maple

The sugar maple is often found on the slopes within the southern parts of North America, and they thrive best where the soils are sandy. They are actually prevalent in the woodlands on hilly areas, and where the hillsides are dry and rocky.

Although this herb does well in different types of soils, they thrive where the soil is rich and properly drained. The best altitude for this plant is from 0 to 1,600 meters above sea level.

The sugar maple has green and sometimes dark green leaves, which gradually become yellow or faded orange. Sometimes the leaves can even turn red, particularly during the fall season.

The plant tends to grow tall, with the full height once mature being between 60 and 75 feet; this height proceeding at an annual rate of between 12 and 24 inches.

The bark of the sugar maple is used to produce some types of compound infusion, which is then applied in droplet form to treat sight problems. The plant sap is particularly effective in the treatment of a sore eye.

Medication produced from the plant's inner section of the bark is a great expectorant, and it is popular as a remedy for coughs. This medication is also said to have health properties that help to cleanse the kidneys, even as it serves as a tonic for the liver. The medication from the bark is often taken in the form of tea.

Milkweed

The milkweed grows in all parts of Canada apart from the north; and within the eastern states of the US. In the US, this herb is particularly prevalent in the prairies, while in Canada it thrives in the southern areas like New Brunswick and Saskatchewan. The milkweed is actually a plant one can easily find growing along the sides of the road or in pastures.

The milkweed grows to a height of a single foot, although some species can reach 6ft. The herb has strong green stems which have tough fibers. It also has narrow leaves, which are long and number around two or three. The flowers of this plant develop in cluster form, and their colors can be clear pink, mellow orange or soft white depending on the particular species.

The milkweed root is rich in medicinal properties. Its sap is credited with treating asthma, coughs and fever. It is also said to be a purgative, and traditionally people would use it to treat kidney stones.

Nettle

The nettle is a plant also known as the stinging nettle; and its scientific name is *Urtica dioica*. It can be found in the US and Canada, and it particularly thrives in soils that are fertile and damp.

The nettle grows as a shrub and develops leaves that are shaped in form of a heart. It also has yellow flowers and sometimes pink ones. The stem of the nettle plant has hairs that are tiny but stiff, and those hairs are responsible for releasing chemicals that sting when someone touches the plant.

The leaves of the plant also have the stinging hairs; and the chemicals produced include histamine and also formic acid. These chemicals not only cause irritation of the skin, but also cause stinging and itching. They also cause redness of the affected skin area.

Herbal medication from the nettle is primarily derived from the leaves, which are brewed in water and drank as a kind of tea. This drink is used for treatment of gout and rheumatism, even as it is used when a person's spleen is abnormally enlarged.

Nettle tea is also credited with having diuretic properties, and also for reducing dysentery.

Oak

The oak is a deciduous tree whose life span is normally in excess of 400 years. This tree thrives very well in North America, where around 90 species of it exist.

The oak tree has a bark with deep ridges as well as fissures that are just as deep. That bark reflects a scaly appearance. The actual colour of the oak bark can range from white-grey to dark-grey, and even black.

The leaves of the oak are pointed and rounded at the tips, and they are also distinctly lobed.

The most potent part of the oak with regard to medicinal properties is the bark. It is credited with producing medicine that can treat infections because of its antiseptic properties, and which also has capacity to treat inflammation and burns.

Herbal medicine from the oak is also used to treat toothaches. It also has hemostatic properties; meaning it can reduce bleeding.

Orange Agoseris

The Orange Agoseris is an herb that belongs to the sunflower species. Sometimes this plant is referred to as the mountain dandelion. It can be found in the western areas of North America, which include states like Alaska and some areas of Canada.

This plant also thrives in the southern areas like California and Arizona, and even New Mexico. Other areas where the orange agoseris exists include the Rocky Mountains, Black Hills, and other areas on the eastern side of the continent. Small quantities of the herb can also be found in the central areas of Quebec, the Otish Mountains and the Chic Choc Mountains.

The orange agoseris, a perennial plant, does not have a stem. Instead, its leaves develop from the base in form of a rosette. The stem-like features this herb produces are peduncles, each of which bears one flower head.

The tiny flowers produced by this plant are usually orange in colour, although sometimes they can be yellow, purple, or even pink or red.

The edible parts of the orange agoseris where medicinal substances can be extracted from are the leaves and the plant flowers. Sometimes people draw sap from the stem, and they combine it with the leaves for chewing; the same way people chew gum. When applied on the external part of the body, the medicine from this herb treats snake bites and bites from insects. It can also treat an abscess or a swelling.

Pasque Flower

The pasque flower can be found in areas of North America, in places like the British Columbia, Ontario, Winnipeg and Manitoba in Canada.

The flowers of this plant have styles that are white in colour, and sometimes they are purple. These are surrounded by stamens in bright yellow. As for the sepals, their colour ranges from a pale purple to dark purple. Still, there are some pasque flowers whose sepals are white.

The medicine from the pasque flower should be diluted significantly before consumption.

It is said to relieve headaches and to treat neuralgia. It is also credited with alleviating what is termed 'nerve exhaustion,' which usually affects women.

The medication from this herb is also used by homeopaths in its very dilute form as treatment for eye ailments and various diseases of the skin. This medication is also credited with alleviating toothache.

Passionflower

The passionflower, whose scientific name is Passiflora incarnate, also goes by the names maypop, wild apricot and purple passionflower. It can be found in North America, and mostly within the southern areas of the US.

The passionflower grows fast and in form of a vine, and its stem is the climbing type. The stem is also smooth and long, and it has several tendrils. This herb produces leaves that have three or five lobes each.

As for the flowers produced by the passionflower, they are purple-blue in colour. The fruits of the passionflower are shaped like an egg, but they are green in colour.

The parts of the passionflower above the ground's surface are edible, including the fruits. These fruits are often termed 'maypops.' The medication derived from these plant parts serves as a sedative, which is generally considered mild. For that reason it is often used to help a person who has problems falling asleep.

Medication from this herb is also used for lowering cholesterol and for treatment of heart ailments and diabetes.

Owing to the fact that passion fruits are rich in minerals such as calcium, folate, and magnesium and others like potassium and phosphorus, they are considered good for enhancing the health of the kidneys, the nerves and the muscles.

Peppermint

The peppermint, whose scientific name is Mentha Canadensis, is mostly found in the north-western areas of North America. In fact, it is sometimes referred to as the Canada mint or American wild mint.

The peppermint plant is perennial, and its height can reach 3ft. It is easy to identify this herb through its scent, and its flowers that are a light purple. Its leaves are green in colour, and they are serrated along the edges.

Peppermint leaves and the oil extracted from peppermint are medicinal. The medicine is said to treat nausea and diarrhea, as well as flatulence and other problems of indigestion. Owing to the calming property of the medication, it has been found to help during menstrual and nerve pains, as well as muscle aches.

Another health condition said to be alleviated by the peppermint herbal medicine is Irritable Bowel Syndrome, abbreviated as IBS.

It is important to note there are different types of mints and not all of them are edible. The way to know an edible mint is by checking its aroma. The edible mints have the aroma of wintergreen; as exemplified by peppermint or spearmint.

Pine

The pine is a tree that belongs to the Pinus species, and it grows in different parts of the world including the eastern part of North America. The tallest type of this plant is found in Maine.

The pine has wood whose grains are tightly bound, and sap that is thick and also white in colour. Its leaves are deciduous and they develop in clusters. This plant has a strong stem whose grains are closely positioned.

The colour of the pine stem is normally dark in colour. The clusters of pine leaves emerge from sheaths and these leaves form two bundles.

Pine needles are used in baths alongside bath salts for relief of headaches and muscle aches. The same combination is used for purposes of soothing headaches and for treatment of skin irritations.

The needle hairs of the pine plant are also used when rinsing hair, for purposes of eliminating dandruff and treating eczema. The rinse is also credited with adding some shine to the hair.

Plantain

The plantain is a plant that originated in Africa, and it grows in the tropical areas of North America when cultivated.

The plantain plant is a banana type that is larger than the ordinary banana. It develops its original colour from green to yellow over time; and sometimes they become a dark brown colour. Plantains have a thick skin.

Plantain's leaves are medicinal, just like the herb's seeds. The medicine has been found to treat ailments of the skin such as dermatitis, inflammation of the skin, bruises, eczema, tiny cuts, and even insect stings and bites.

Prickly Pear

The prickly pear belongs to the family of cactuses. It thrives in areas of North America like New Mexico, Montana, Florida, Massachusetts and even in Ontario.

A prickly pear has spines and flowers that are very beautiful. In fact, the beauty of these flowers has inspired poets in their art. These flowers are very distinct because they grow on pears that are prickly. The flowers of prickly pears have many stamens and thin sepals.

The parts of the prickly pear that are edible include its leaves and flowers, as well as its stem and fruit. The prickly pear needs to be boiled first, or grilled, before it can be consumed.

The medicine from this herb has been found to treat diabetes and to lower cholesterol. It is also credited with helping reduce obesity and to fight hangovers.

It is also said this herb has anti-viral properties, as well as capacity to fight inflammation.

Evening Primrose

The evening primrose grows naturally in different areas of North America; which include the states of Missouri and Nebraska, Oklahoma and Kansas, and even in Texas. It is one of those plants that thrive in areas whose soils are not fertile and where moisture is minimal and the sun hot.

The evening primrose grows to a height of between eighteen and twenty-four inches. It produces flowers that are pink in colour, and which are sometimes white or pale lavender; hence the herb is described as being showy.

The primrose herb as a whole is medicinal; meaning its roots, seeds, leaves and even the flower buds and the blossoms have healing properties.

The plant oil, popularly known as the evening primrose oil, abbreviated as EPO, is in widespread use. Its potency is mostly associated with the GLA or gamma-linolenic acid it has, which is actually a fatty acid of the Omega-6 type.

Owing to the abundance of EPO, the oil is effective when used to treat skin problems like clearance of acne, and other conditions like eczema. The oil is also credited with reducing breast pain when a woman is menstruating, and can even stop hot flashes.

The presence of linolenic acid gives the oil capacity to reduce nerve pains and even pains emanating from the bones.

Native Americans also used the herb medicine for treatment of bruises and haemorrhoids.

Purslane

The purslane can be found in North America, especially in the state of California. It also does well in areas where the altitude is 4,600ft; areas that are normally used for agricultural purposes.

The purslane has the tendency to grow fast during the spring season and also summer. The purslane plant spreads like a mat as it grows, and while its height goes to 6 inches, the mat-like spread goes up to 2 feet.

The stem of the purslane is round and thick and also succulent. Its colour can be light green, but it can also be a brownish-red. The leaves of this herb whose colour is a glossy green also turn purplish-red over time. They also develop in form of a cluster close to the tip of the stem.

The purslane herb has several medicinal parts, including its leaves, seeds and stem, as well as its flower buds.

The medication derived from this herb has purgative properties, and it also serves as a tonic for cardiac issues. It is also used for relaxation of muscles and as an emollient. It also fights inflammation and has diuretic properties.

Medicine from the purslane herb is also credited with fighting osteoporosis as well as psoriasis.

Red Clover

The red clover can be found in North America, especially in areas like Hawaii and even in Alaska.

The red clover is found in spaces within forests, as well as along the forest edges, as long as the areas are beneath 8,500ft.

The red clover has flowers with round heads that comprise several flowerets that are tubular in shape.

The medicinal parts of the red clover herb include the plant flowers and its leaves. They can be consumed either fresh or in dried form.

This plant, which has Vitamins B and C, is very rich in protein; and it has capacity to treat serious ailments like whooping cough and others of a respiratory nature.

It can also treat inflammations of the skin like eczema and psoriasis.

Redroot

The red root can be found in the plains along the Atlantic coast, particularly in Canada. This herb thrives very well in the southern parts of Nova Scotia.

The red root is a perennial herb that develops a rhizome close to the surface of the earth. It has an upright stem and produces sap that is red in colour. One distinct feature of this plant's stem is that it has no branches. It also grows to a height that is between 15 and 40 centimeters.

This stem has a whitish colour in its young stages, but as it matures the colour turns tawny.

The leaves of the red root are boiled for purposes of making a form of tea, which is then used for treatment. Nevertheless, the entire plant has medicinal properties, and extracts from any part of it can be used to prepare herbal medicine.

Medication from this herb is often used as treatment for colds and fever as well as pneumonia. It has also been found to treat UTIs or urinary tract infections, and ailments of a digestive nature. It is also said to diminish toothaches.

Romero

The Romero Rosemary whose name was derived from Latin means 'dew of the sea.' It can be found in North America, especially along the lakeshores in the southern areas of Nova Scotia. The herb is actually mostly prevalent in Canada, and more so along the Atlantic coast.

The Rosemary has aromatic leaves that produce a taste that is both tangy and bitter once they have been dried. At the same time, they produce a flavour whose fragrance is pine-like. It is actually this flavour that makes it very popular for culinary purposes.

The Romero, or Rosemary herb, has medicinal leaves. Also, oil is extracted from the plant for use as an herbal treatment.

The leaves are used in cooking and their healing effect is received by consuming the food. The treatment here includes solving digestive problems and heartburn, as well as diminishing intestinal gas. It also includes improvement of appetite, and alleviation of other health problems like those linked to the gall bladder and the liver.

Sagebrush

The sagebrush is also termed the 'big sagebrush,' and it can be found in North America in states like California, Colorado, Dakota and British Columbia. It is also found within New Mexico's western side of the Great Plains.

Although the shrub that is the sagebrush is dominant in the Great Basin of North America, it also exists in cold deserts and in areas where soils are sandy or powdery. It is also found in riparian lands where the sagebrush touches the green zone.

The leaves of the sagebrush are hairy and grey in colour, and they normally grow to a length of one inch. They are also shaped like a wedge, and each leaf has 3 teeth at its end.

Once the leaf of a sagebrush is crushed, it releases a spicy smell that is also bitter; and so it is easy to tell if an area is dominated by sagebrush if such a smell can be detected.

The sagebrush has stems that are grey in colour just like its twigs, and in its early days the twigs have hairs. As they mature, those twigs develop a weak bark that can fall off with ease.

The leaves, seed and the fruit of the sagebrush are all edible. Medicine made from them has capacity to treat wounds and stop internal bleeding. The medication is also said to treat colds and fight headaches.

BOOK 2

NATIVE AMERICAN
HERBAL APOTHECARY

CHAPTER 1

HOW TO SOURCE HERBS & PREPARE THEM

Herbs meant to be used for medicinal purposes can be harvested from their natural habitats, and they can also be grown like other food crops.

One of the oldest methods of collecting herbs is referred to as wildcrafting. Whether you are getting the plants for medicinal purposes or just for food, the method of attaining these herbs is called wildcrafting.

A major benefit of wildcrafting is that the herbs you find are comparatively richer in nutrients and medicinal potency because of growing in a natural environment. Some of those areas have not been disturbed for a long time, and so they continue getting richer in nutrients. Another factor that contributes to the richness of plants from the wild is they grow amidst several other plant species.

From the ancient days when Native Americans relied a lot on natural foods for sustenance and natural medicine for treatment, wildcrafting has been helped to keep a good environmental balance.

As people harvest the herbs at the time of need, they leave others to continue to grow and mature, to be used at a later date. Wildcrafting, done responsibly, is great at pruning plants that need sufficient room to expand, as well as leaving enough room to attain the sunlight they need.

It also helps that people take the opportunity to remove dried parts that are unhelpful to the plants. In short, in wildcrafting, the natural habitat benefits even as people who consume the plants do.

At the same time, whether purposefully or incidentally, new plants are planted as people do their business around the bushes and forests, and so plant growth is continuous.

Best Techniques of Sourcing Herbs from the Wild

There are different ways of sourcing plants from where they grow naturally, but it is important that only the best techniques are used. This is important for the purpose of ensuring that natural bushes and forests are not depleted.

By best technique is meant the methods that ensure both the herb users and the environment can continue to benefit from human activity. If the methods used are inappropriate, where people harvest herbs without concern as to what happens to the environment, soon future generations could be unable to find natural herbs to use for either food or natural healing.

Harvesting Shrubby Plants

If the plant you want for your medicine is a shrub and the part you want is either a branch or the stem, ensure the spot you aim to cut is above a leaf node. This is crucial because from that leaf node will emerge another branch or stem; and the plant continues to thrive.

The distance from the node to the spot you aim to slice should be 6 millimeters apart; and your cut should be at an angle of 45°. The only time you may cut right across is if the plant you are getting your piece of herb from has two leaves exactly opposite each other on that spot.

Replanting

Whenever you harvest an herb, pick its root crown and replant it whenever that is possible.

Timing

If you intend to source your herbal medicine from a root, make a point of harvesting your roots during the fall season. The reason for this is that it is during fall that leaves drop off their mother plants; or they simply die. When this happens, the bulk of nutrients end up within the plant's roots.

Not only are you bound to harvest potent roots, but any remaining roots are likely to continue becoming strong faster.

Starting with Broken Branches

If there are any branches that are broken and hanging off the plant, harvest those first. By so doing, you will have accomplished your mission of getting herbs for use, and beyond that you will have protected the plant from possible infection.

So, to reduce the chances of the plant developing a disease, cut off that broken branch in a manner that flattens the broken surface.

How to Cut a Branch Safely

If you want to cut off a tree branch, ensure to begin by cutting it into a depth of two inches on its underside. Only after that can you continue to saw the branch from the usual top side.

The reason for this is that while the bark of the tree is safe at the top surface because you continue sawing deep into the tree, you run the risk of peeling off the bark on the underside if you do not have a ready cut beneath.

In short, you want to cut off the branch you need for your use but leave the tree with its bark intact; and not partly stripped.

How to Gather Medicinal Herbs

It is important to understand the dos and don'ts of wildcrafting, where wildcrafting stands for harvesting of herbal plants from their natural habitat for medicinal use.

Native Americans and people from other ancient cultures carried out wildcrafting in their time, and used the plants as sources of medicine and also as important ingredients during particular rituals.

Although these uses have continued for many centuries, there are still medicinal herbs available for use in forests and bushes; the reason being that the people concerned have continued their herb harvesting in a responsible manner.

It is, therefore, important to learn how best to go about harvesting herbs for medicinal use, so these herbs do not become extinct. It would, undoubtedly, be great if future generations can benefit from herb-based natural treatments the way others before them have done.

Spare endangered plants

First of all, make a point of sparing any species of herb you know to be endangered. This will help it to flourish and be available for use sometime in the future.

Identify plants correctly

Identify the plant correctly before proceeding to harvest it. One reason for this is that you run the risk of consuming a poisonous herb if you mistakenly pick the wrong plant. Some herbs resemble one another, and it only takes one or two features, sometimes inconspicuous, to differentiate them.

Another reason is that if you pick the herb you did not intend to, you probably will end up discarding it; and that will be an unnecessary waste.

Avoid the highly placed plants

There is good reason to avoid the plants on very high ground, which are usually far more mature than the rest – repopulation.

Often you will be harvesting your herbs from land that is slanting and rising in gradient as you move up. Once you avoid moving to the peak, you let those mature plants drop seeds to areas below where more herbs can continue growing. In short, the herb harvesting area should be somewhere below the top areas where mature plants are mostly established.

Only pick where there is abundance

If from a given herb species you want to harvest some branches, choose the plants with several healthy branches. This is because it is important you leave the plant strong and healthy, and in a position to produce more branches and to continue thriving.

You should do the same if you are targeting leaves as well. It is important that you leave the plant with sufficient leaves to make food for the plant and to play the other roles plant leaves do within the habitat.

One important principle you need to adhere to is ensuring that what you pick from a single plant does not exceed 10% of what that plant has.

Best Time to Pick Herbs

Every part of the plant has its appropriate harvesting time. If these periods are adhered to, all the parts of the plants will continue to develop well and to thrive, so that procreation continues without interference.

Flower Harvesting

If you want to source your herbal medicine from flowers, the best time to pick these is when they start blooming. As for the best time of day, this should be from 6 a.m. to 10 a.m.

Leaf Harvesting

If you want to use plant leaves for your natural medicine, the best time to pick these is prior to the plants starting to flower. As for the best time of day, this should also be done from 6 a.m. to 10 a.m.

Root Harvesting

The best time to harvest herbal roots is after the plant has passed the seeding period. As for the timing, early morning is best because then the affected soil is unlikely to become too dry soon after. For plants that are biannual, harvesting is discouraged during the plant's first year of life. For, the plant's second year, the best time to harvest herbs is in autumn.

Bark Harvesting

The best period to harvest bark is in the spring. Even then, it is advised that bark should not be stripped from the entire length of the branch or tree. In short, whatever bark the tree has should only be removed partially and in an appropriate manner.

Another point to note is that the branch you choose for bark harvesting ought to be reasonably far from the ground. The reason for this precaution is that if you harvest bark from a branch close to the earth's surface, the part you leave naked will be at risk of fungal infection; and subsequent rot.

As you do your bark harvesting, it is recommended that you target the inner area of the bark for extraction of medicine. This inner part is referred to as the cambium.

At the same time, it is recommended that you make a point of pollarding, which means cutting off the tip of the tree and the ends of branches for the purpose of enhancing growth toward the top areas. Pollarding is most recommended for branches that are short.

Another recommendation targets those tree stumps that are short; and it involves coppicing. By this is meant the practice of cutting down the stump up to the earth's surface; the purpose being to stimulate fresh growth.

Harvesting of Sap & Pitch

These two, sap and the plant pitch, are best harvested toward the end of winter; if not, then in the early days of spring. Pitch in this case is that plant polymer that is visco-elastic in nature, and which is alternatively referred to as resin.

Harvesting of Fruits & Seeds

The best time to harvest fruit or even seeds for medicinal purposes is when they have fully matured.

How to Farm Medicinal Herbs

If the methods used for farming medicinal herbs are appropriate, both the wild animals and the people who need herbs will have enough to use. One way of ensuring natural habitats have sufficient vegetation is to avoid harvesting from the same location every year. Nevertheless, the area needs to be cared for all through.

Among the actions you need to take to ensure the herbs are well tended is thinning. This involves removing some flowers, or even young fruits, in order that those that remain develop faster.

Thinning also helps to avoid a situation where one place is so densely populated with plants that flowering becomes a problem.

Another important action you need to take whenever necessary is root separation. This involves division of plants by digging up whole clumps and thereafter dividing the crown as well as the root ball. The divisions can be two or numerous, dependent how big an individual clump is.

Top pinching is something else you need to do as part of the process of tending the plant habitat. By pinching is meant a pruning technique meant for encouraging plants to develop several branches as opposed to just one shoot.

For example, if a plant is pinched off at its tip, it is likely to stop growing farther upward. Instead, other branches begin to shoot off the stem of the plant below the spot where the pinching off was done.

It is also crucial that people protect any surviving older plants for the sake of continuity of growth. These plants are great facilitators of such continuity because they readily produce seeds. Their other crucial role in the habitat is protection of young plants, which might otherwise be destroyed by natural elements such as excessive sunlight or strong raindrops.

Whatever action you take in the wild, ensure it does not introduce or exacerbate the risk of soil erosion. One way of diminishing such risk is replanting herbs, especially if you have been harvesting plant roots. Also, it is helpful to fill up any spaces dug up, and to avoid leaving potholes behind.

It is recommended that you make a point of introducing new plants on hilly areas you find cleared. If other parts of the environment have excess foliage lying around, you could gather some and scatter it on bare areas.

When working on a hilly area, avoid shoes with hard soles because they could cause serious harm to the ecosystems within the area, particularly if these ecosystems are fragile.

How to Harvest, Store and Dry herbs

For best management of herbs and their sources, it is important that proper harvesting habits are formed and the herbs well preserved. It is crucial that you do not affect the roots as you pull off the herb's leaves.

Plant Parts above Ground

If the parts of the plant you want to harvest are above ground surface, the best time for harvesting is from 6 a.m. to 10 a.m. This is the period just before these herbs begin to wilt.

When harvesting flowers, check to see that the bud is about to bloom; which you can establish from the bud's colour. Generally, the best time to harvest parts of the herbs above ground surface is during or immediately following the full moon.

Plant Roots

The best period to harvest herb roots is after the plant has produced its seeds. Timing should ideally be early morning before the rising of the sun.

Tree Barks

The best period to harvest tree barks is during spring or autumn. When it comes to bark harvesting, in case the plant population is dense, it is acceptable to pull out entire plants. However, it is important that thinning be done instead of clearing whole bushes, ensuring the trees that are left are healthy.

Best Herb Drying Techniques

Most herbs need to be dried under the shade and in a place with good ventilation. It is also to establish if the herbs you have are better dried in sunshine.

It is also recommended that herbs and flowers are not washed. Nevertheless, these should be shaken so that if there are any pests attached to the herbs, or even dirt, these can drop off.

One technique of drying herbs involves tying them up first into bundles, the diameter of each bundle being 1.5 inches or below, when the stem base area is measured.

Another drying technique is spreading individual herbs on your windows.

If the part of the plant you want to dry is the bark, it is recommended that you peel off its outer part; this move being termed as tossing.

When drying roots, you need to spread them out; if not, dry them after looping them. It should be remembered it is important to clean dirt from the roots, and although rinsing or brushing with hands may be effective in cleaning some roots, it may be difficult to be thorough in some cases, especially where the roots have grown in clay.

Where the dirt is tough to get off, it is advisable to use a pressure hose to clean the roots off.

In case the roots you want to dry are broad or thick, you need to slice them lengthwise as long as these roots are not the aromatic type. If they are the aroma may escape or be adversely affected.

Safe Herb Storage

Store your harvested herbs in a place where there is no direct or excessive light. There should not be any heat either. If these elements are present, they may destroy any aroma the herbs have.

If the herbs are going to be kept unused for a long time, the best way to preserve them is to secure them in the plastic bags used to preserve food. You can also store them safely in fiber barrels. In the absence of food grade bags or fiber barrels, you can store your herbs in any container that keeps out oxygen and moisture.

Appropriate storage not only ensures the herbs remain dry, but that their potency remains consistent all through. It is also crucial to note that whenever possible you should leave your herbs whole; meaning you should avoid dicing or slicing them. This is because when broken or entirely crushed, herbs lose their value faster.

The final act in storage preparation should entail correctly labelling and dating every herb package. This means you can easily identify whatever herb you want to use.

CHAPTER 2

HOW TO PREPARE HERBAL MEDICATIONS

Many of the herbs you harvest are meant to provide medications in varying forms, such as decoctions, tinctures and others. You, therefore, need to know how to go about preparing the medications in their different forms.

How to Prepare Herbal Infusions

Herbal infusion is the same as herbal tea. To prepare an herbal infusion, all you need to do is pour boiling water onto the herbs; whether those herbs are fresh or are in dried form.

The parts of the plant that are usually infused are those that are soft; which is mostly the leaves or the plant's flowers.

It is from this process of infusion that you derive green tea, black tea, and such other herbal teas.

The ratio of ingredients when you want to make green tea is normally a teaspoonful of herbs in their dried state to one cup of hot water.

When you want to prepare black tea, the ratio of ingredients is normally 4 teaspoonfuls of herbs in their dried state to a cup of hot water.

How to Prepare Herbal Decoctions

An herbal decoction is the liquid made when you put herbs in water and then simmer or boil the mixture. Plant parts that are mostly used to prepare decoctions are the tough ones; and they include the plant's stems, seeds, barks and roots.

During the boiling process, the potent part of the herb, which happens to be soluble in water, seeps into the water; and that is how the decoction is created. A good example of an herbal decoction is garlic soup.

To prepare garlic soup, put a teaspoonful of dried garlic into one cup of water, and then let the mixture simmer.

If you want to use fresh garlic, put 4 teaspoonfuls of garlic in one cup of water, and then let the mixture simmer.

For either the dried herb or the fresh one, the simmering should last 5 minutes. Thereafter you need to strain the mixture and it will be ready for use.

How to Prepare Herbal Percolations

Percolation is that process followed to prepare drinks such as coffee. So, when using percolation to prepare herbs, you need to put in herbs that have been ground in something like a sieve or piece of cloth, and then run water, or even alcohol, through that mass of powdered herbs.

How to Prepare Herbal Tincture

To prepare herbal tincture, all you need to do is chop herbs, put them in a blender and then add alcohol. When you blend or macerate that mixture, your resulting product is an herbal tincture.

It is important to know there are alternatives to alcohol. For example, apple cider can be used, and glycerin can also be used in place of alcohol.

You can, for instance, chop echinacea flowers into tiny pieces when they are still fresh, put them in a blender, and then add your solvent of choice. Then proceed with your maceration process.

Ordinarily your ingredients ratio when making a tincture is 1:5, where an ounce of ground herb is mixed with 5 ounces of liquid.

After your blending, you need to put your mixture in the refrigerator for a period of 4hrs, after which you can strain it. For storage purposes, you can put your tincture in a bottle.

How to do Double Extraction

The process of double extraction involves carrying out two extraction processes that are almost similar. You begin by extracting what you want from the herb by first passing alcohol or heated water through the herb material.

Next you focus on the herb remnants, and you extract its richness in a similar manner. Finally, you take both liquids and mix them; forming what is termed as dual extract.

In a practical herb preparation situation, what you need to do is take your chosen herb, dry it and grind it into powder form. Pour the mixture in a container that you can cover and refrigerate; and then let it rest for some days. In fact, you can keep it for as long as two weeks.

If you do not want to use your refrigerator you can cover your mixture nicely and store it in a dark section of your cupboard.

Note that you need to keep shaking the mixture two times a day for the duration of storage. After the duration of rest, the next step is straining of the mixture using a sieve, making a point of squeezing the remnants left in the sieve. The idea is to collect every drop possible from the herb mixture. Up to this stage the process is referred to as single extraction, and what you have prepared is an herbal tincture.

For double extraction to be accomplished, put the herb mash that is the remnant in the sieve in some container and add water into it. Put the mixture on fire and let it simmer for half an hour. After that you need to sieve that mixture; and now you will have prepared a decoction.

The final step involves mixing the tincture with the decoction; hence completing your double extraction.

BOOK 3

NATIVE AMERICAN HERBAL REMEDIES

CHAPTER 1

IMPORTANCE OF INCORPORATING HERBS INTO REGULAR DIET

Herbs are potent with healing properties, whether you choose to extract the medicinal part for use, or whether you consume the herb as part of your food ingredients. Many herbs are known for their culinary value, and many people only come to realize later they are also medicinal.

When the European settlers arrived in North America, they were very impressed with the health and overall strength of the Native Americans. They not only found these natives full of beauty, but they also found them to be strong and brave. The Europeans were also amazed at how alert these Native Americans seemed to be at all times.

There is also historical evidence from archaeologists that confirms these Native Americans had great physical fortitude; having none of the modern day bone deficiencies, teeth cavities, and other serious health conditions.

It has also been established that while the known diseases among the Native Americans during those early days were 87, today the number of diseases that make the list of those known in North America is in excess of 30,000.

Another outstanding fact regarding the ancient people's way of life is that the Native American women were remarkably strong. They would give birth without assistance, and take an extremely short time off before resuming their normal day-to-day work routine.

This extraordinary health status witnessed in Native Americans is attributed to their daily diet. They relied mainly on whole natural foods, primarily dominated by herbs.

Although herbs were used to treat diseases, these were often the mild ones or those that occurred by accident; i.e. common cold, cuts, insect bites, snake bites, sprains, and such other unforeseeable illnesses. Serious diseases that are prevalent today, like bronchitis, tuberculosis, diabetes, high blood pressure and such others were rare or non-existent.

This is because the herbs the people used in their daily food served to prevent such illnesses. Also, any signs of disease were dealt with through herbs, and the chances of a mild illness developing into a serious one were curtailed.

For example, when someone caught a common cold, herbal tea was made from the rose hip herb or even from pine needles, and the person would drink it as treatment. The same was done when someone caught the flu.

These Native Americans were very knowledgeable about specific herbs and what they could treat, but they could not explain the reason the particular herbs were effective remedies.

Modern scientific information has revealed the components in each of the herbs used, and so today it is possible to explain why certain foods are best included in people's daily diet.

For example, the herbs used to fight colds, like the pine needles, are rich in Vitamin C as well as bioflavonoids, and these are the active ingredients that treat colds. Other herbs contain elements that bear pertinent healing properties; and these elements include Phyto-chemicals, enzymes and vitamins, and even minerals.

When these medicinal herbs are included in people's diet, they enhance the immunity of the body, making it strong enough to ward off illnesses.

Next, you are going to learn the healing powers important herb elements have; and why the herbs help to keep diseases at bay when incorporated into people's daily diet.

The Effect of Phyto-chemicals

For starters, 'Phyto' stands for plant; and so Phyto-chemicals simply means the chemicals within plants. It is possible to isolate these Phyto-chemicals when they are found in a plant in high concentrations.

While some of the natural chemicals found in herbs are anti-oxidants great in fighting cancer, others are effective in lowering the level of cholesterol, reducing plaque that layer the arteries, and also stimulating the immune system. They are also effective in stimulating production of enzymes. Next are explanations on the effect of various Phyto-chemicals.

Importance of Alkaloids

Alkaloids are nitrogenous compounds of an organic nature, found in herbs such as the goldenseal. Once consumed, it ensures the yeast in the body does not exceed the normal level. Effectively, therefore, when people incorporate foods rich in alkaloids into their diet, the bacteria the body needs are maintained at a healthy level. Maintenance of such healthy bacterial levels is particularly crucial in the gastro-intestinal tract as well as the urinary tract. This bacterial status is also a boost to the immune system.

Importance of Anthocyanidins

Anthocyanidins belong to the category of Phyto-chemicals found in raspberries, bilberries, and black currants.

Their effectiveness in treatment comes from the capacity they have of fighting free radicals, which are unhealthy by-products of the body's metabolic reaction. If uncontrolled, free radicals can cause illnesses of a degenerative nature in the body, such as diseases of the heart or even cancer.

Anthocyanidins are also effective in mitigating formation of plaque in the blood vessels and enhancing flow of blood in the body; minimizing the risk of cardiovascular ailments; fighting of inflammation; improving vision; and even inhibiting edema. The term 'edema' stands for any swelling formed as a result of accumulated fluid.

Importance of Chlorophyll

Chlorophyll is that green pigment that every green plant has. It is credited with fighting bacteria, hastening healing of wounds and even burns, and helping to fight cancer. It also contains Vitamin K, which helps in clotting of blood and in enhancing the health of bones.

The Importance of Diterpenes

Diterpenes are present in several herbs, one of those herbs being rosemary. They are chemical compounds with anti-oxidant properties. They also help to fight cancer and to eliminate toxins from the liver.

The Importance of Eleutherosides

Eleutherosides are found in the roots of the Siberian ginseng, whose botanical name is Eleutherococcus senticosus; other times simply known as eleuthero. These chemical compounds have been known for their effectiveness in increasing stamina, stimulating appetite, and enhancing mental energy.

Eleutherosides are also credited with stimulating body metabolism, strengthening immunity, and also stimulating the CNS or Central Nervous System. They have also been found to regularize the menstrual cycle and to dissipate hot flashes.

The Importance of Essential Fatty Acids

The Omega 3 and 6 fats that comprise the essential fatty acids are necessary for the health of the body, yet the body does not generate them. As such, the body benefits immensely when herbs with these essential fatty acids are incorporated into a person's daily diet.

One of the crucial roles of these fats is maintaining cell membranes' integrity, and that of the nerve fibers' protective cover.

Another of these fats' important roles is stimulating production of prostaglandins, important substances that resemble hormones, and which help to reduce the level of cholesterol and to enhance immunity.

The Importance of Flavonglycosides

Herbs with flavonglycosides are very helpful in the body as flavonglycosides are very potent as anti-oxidants; meaning they can easily eliminate free radicals. Flavonglycosides are also capable of dilating blood vessels and enhancing the flow of blood in the body. They also have capacity to enhance mental clearness and vision, as well as hearing. One of the herbs rich in flavonglycosides is Ginkgo biloba.

The Importance of Gingerols

Herbs with gingerols are beneficial in the diet as they have anti-oxidant properties. Gingerols also help in enhancement of the digestive function where proteins are concerned; and also with regards to fat.

Gingerols are also important in the diet as they contributing to soothing of the stomach and elimination of toxicity from the liver. They also help to reduce liver inflammation. One of the herbs rich in gingerols is ginger.

The Importance of Ginkolic Acid

Any herb with ginkolic acid has anti-oxidant properties, as ginkolic acid is essentially an anti-oxidant. Ginkolic acid is also renowned for its capacity to enhance blood circulation as well as mental clarity. Other important properties of this anti-oxidant include fighting depression and preventing cancer.

The Importance of Glycyrrhizins

Glycyrrhizins are Phyto-chemicals found in herbs such as the licorice, which protect the body from viral attacks and inflammation. They also have capacity to protect the skin and to inhibit formation of tumors.

The Importance of Hypericin

Hypericin is effective in mood enhancement, and so it keeps people in high spirits when they incorporate herbs rich with it; like St. John's Wort. The way hypericin is thought to work is through regulation of the brain's neurotransmitters.

The Importance of Isothiocyanates

Isothiocyanates are Phyto-chemicals present in herbs like the horseradish; and they have capacity to catalyze generation of protective enzymes. They also have the potential of inhibiting damage to a person's DNA; which means that herbs rich in isothiocyanates, when incorporated in the daily diet, can reduce the risk of developing cancer of the breasts.

The Importance of Lactones

Lactones are important in that they help in fighting cancer. Consuming foods that have lactones, such as the root from the kava kava herb, ensures any harmful carcinogens are expelled from the body. As a result, your risk of developing cancer is reduced.

The Importance of Lipoic Acid

Lipoic acid is one of those Phyto-chemicals present in several plants. It is a strong anti-oxidant with the potential to expel any heavy metals that may have entered your body. Lipoic acid is also credited with regulating the level of glucose in the blood, protecting the body from heart ailments, and fighting cancer. Also, when you consume foods with lipoic acid, your energy level is enhanced.

The Importance of Phenolic Acid

Phenolic acids have anti-oxidant properties known for inhibiting formation of agents with potential to cause cancer. Herbs rich in phenolic acids include berries and parsley. They can also be found in other flowering herbs in varying concentrations.

The Importance of Phthalides

Phthalides are other Phyto-chemicals beneficial to human health when incorporated in the diet. It plays its role by catalyzing generation of enzymes that are crucial for a person's general health; and also by getting rid of carcinogens that would otherwise harm the body. An example of an herb rich in phthalides is parsley.

The Importance of Polyacetylenes

Polyacetylenes are great at protecting the body against harmful carcinogens, and also in regulating generation of prostaglandins. Parsley serves as an example of an herb rich in polyacetylenes.

The Importance of Proanthocyanins

The Phyto-chemicals, proanthocyanins, have anti-oxidant properties. They protect the body so it does not develop cancer, and at the same time regulates the level of cholesterol.

Proanthocyanins are also credited with fighting the influenza-causing virus, and strengthening the walls of the blood vessels.

Among the herbs rich in proanthocyanins are elderberries and bilberries.

The Importance of Quercetin

Quercetin is among the phyto-chemicals known as flavanoids, and it is present in very many plants. It has anti-oxidant properties and also acts as an anti-histamine. It also has anti-inflammatory properties and helps to fight cancer.

Quercetin also has capacity to stabilize the membranes of body cells, and also to strengthen capillaries so they do not become too fragile.

Like many flavanoids, quercetin is present in several of the fruits and vegetables commonly consumed.

The Importance of Rosemarinic Acid

Rosemarinic acid, which is rosemary's active portion, is known for fighting nausea and intestinal gas, and solving digestion-related problems in general. It is also credited with fighting headaches.

The Importance of Salin

Salin, also referred to as salicin, is known for fighting inflammation, relieving pain, and even fighting fever. It is also credited with fighting the influenza-causing virus. The white willow is one herb very rich in salin, which is normally extracted from the plant's bark.

The Importance of Saponins

Saponins are among the phyto-chemicals with capacity to fight cancer. They are also credited with fighting inflammation and fungal infections, as well as hastening healing of wounds. They also have anti-bacterial properties and help to lower cholesterol levels.

Among the herbs rich in saponins are licorice and yucca, as well as black cohosh. The ginseng plant also, particularly its root, has saponins in abundance.

The Importance of Silymarin

The phyto-chemical, silymarin is rich in anti-oxidant properties, and it is especially known for protecting the liver. One of the herbs richest in silymarin is the milk thistle.

The Importance of Tannins

The phyto-chemicals known as tannins have anti-oxidant and anti-viral properties. They are also credited with strengthening of the blood capillaries, fighting heart disease as well as asthma, and helping the body resist cancer.

The Importance of Terpenes

Terpenes, the phyto-chemicals popularly referred to as monoterpenes, have anti-oxidant properties. Like all herbs with anti-oxidant properties, herbs rich in terpenes are great at eliminating free radicals from the body. A good example of an herb rich in terpenes is ginkgo biloba.

The Importance of Triterpenoids

Triterpenoids are phyto-chemicals known for the capacity to protect the body from ulcers and even cancer; and to clear the liver of toxicity. They are also credited with protecting teeth from decay.

Herbs particularly rich in triterpenoids include licorice root and gotu kola.

The Role of Enzymes in Healing

As long as an herb has been secured in a place away from intense heat and alcohol, it is bound to have its enzymes intact. Enzymes play a great role in activating the phyto-chemicals as well as all other nutrients present within the herbs.

Enzymes also help the body to process and absorb the herb nutrients consumed, ascertaining these nutrients are biologically available for use.

In order to reap optimal benefits from any herbs consumed, if they have been exposed to extreme heat, it is advisable to take some enzyme supplements alongside the meal. The reason is that exposing herbs to elevated temperatures destroys the enzymes originally available in these herbs.

The kind of supplements recommended are those with proteases, lipases and amylases; meaning those that help in the processing and absorption of proteins, fats, and carbohydrates respectively.

CHAPTER 2

POPULAR HERBAL NATIVE AMERICAN HERBS & THEIR CORRESPONDING REMEDIES

There are very many herbs available in North America, and while some of them are preserved as natural supplements, a number of the popular ones are still consumed raw in the US.

Here we are going to learn here about seven herbs popular in the United States, alongside their common uses.

Ginseng, Garlic, Echinacea & Others

The ginseng herb, whose scientific name is panax quinequefolius, is very popular in the US. In olden days, this herb was popular among many Native American tribes among them the Cherokee and Delaware, who used it as an expectorant to treat fevers, rheumatism, and other serious illnesses like asthma and tuberculosis.

Today, ginseng herb is most popular for its capacity to boost immunity and eliminate stress. The ginseng herb belongs to the family of plants known as araliaceae.

Garlic

Garlic is another herb very popular in the US; and its scientific name is allium sativum. This herb was widely used by the Native Americans, particularly the Cherokee tribe.

They particularly liked garlic for its stimulating effect, and also for its carminative and diuretic properties. This herb, which belongs to the liliaceae family, was also popular among the native tribes because it would serve as an expectorant, treat scurvy and keep worms at bay.

Today, garlic is liked because it lowers cholesterol and enhances cardiovascular wellness.

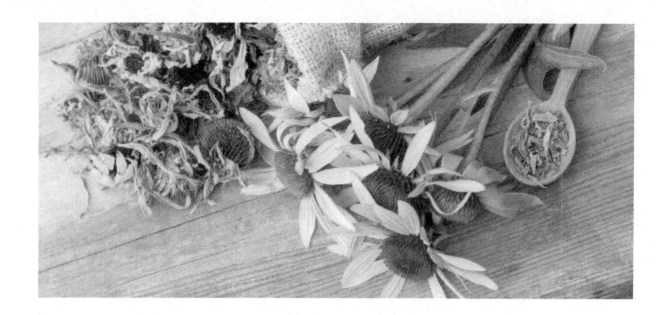

ECHINACEA

Echinacea, scientifically known variously as **Echinacea purpurea** or **Echinacea angustifolia**; or even **Echinacea pallida**, belongs to the **Asteraceae Family**.

The Native American tribes that liked the Echinacea herb very much included the Cheyenne and the Dakota, the Omaha and the Montana, and many others.

They would use the Echinacea to relieve pain and to treat coughs, sore throat and fever; and other ailments like rheumatism, arthritis, mumps and measles; and even smallpox. The Native Americans also used this herb as an antidote whenever poison or any venom was involved.

In modern day, the Echinacea is popular for it capacity to boost immunity.

Goldenseal

The scientific name for goldenseal is hydrastis Canadensis. It is an herb that the Cherokee, the Micmac and the Iroquois Native American tribes particularly liked. They would use the herb to treat fever, pneumonia and whooping cough.

Today, this herb that belongs to the ranunculaceae family, is popular owing to its capacity to boost immunity.

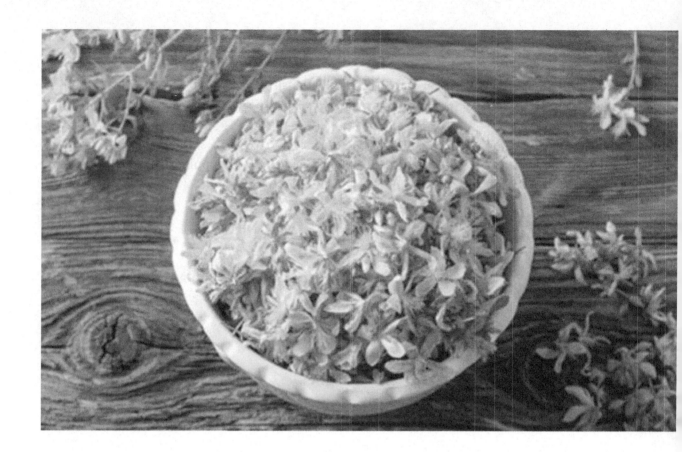

ST. JOHN'S WORT

The scientific name for St. John's Wort is **hypericum perforatum**. It used to be popular among Native American tribes like the Cherokee and the Iroquois, as well as among the Montagnais.

These tribes would use the herb to treat bowel issues, and also fever and coughs.

Today, St. John's Wort, which belongs to the **Hyperiaceae Family**, is popularly used as an antidepressant.

Evening Primrose

The scientific name for the evening primrose is oenothera biennis. This herb, which was very popular among some Native American tribes like the Cherokee and the Ojibwa, and also the Iroquois and the Potawatomi, belongs to the onagraceae family.

These tribes used the herb to alleviate pre-menstrual as well as menstrual discomforts and pain, and pain in the bowels. They also used it to treat obesity.

Present day uses of the evening primrose include alleviation of pre-menstrual as well as menstrual discomfort and pain. The herb is also popular due to its anti-oxidant properties.

Cranberry

The scientific name for the cranberry is vaccinium macrocarpon. It is an herb under the ericaceae family, and which was very popular among the Montagnais tribe, one of the Native American tribes.

These Native Americans used the herb because it would inhibit pain occurring during breathing in cases of pneumonia, or in cases of other chest related ailments. In short, they would consume the herb to treat pleurisy.

In the present day, the cranberry herb is primarily used to treat illnesses associated with the urinary tract.

It is important to note that there are some herb species used in North America for their healing properties, are also prevalent in different regions of the globe. Good examples are the Sambucus nigra, commonly known as the European elderberry or the black elder; Sambucus racemosa, otherwise called the red elderberry; and the Juniperus communis, commonly known as juniper.

As for the black elder, the Native Americans would dry its berries and then use them to make juice, and that juice would serve as treatment for influenza, headache, dental and nerve aches, sciatica and infections. They would also use that black elder juice as either as a diuretic or laxative.

Native Americans would use the red elderberry for its emetic properties; meaning its capacity to trigger vomiting.

As for the medicinal value the Native Americans attached to the juniper herb, it serves as contraceptive for the women.

Other herbs were indigenous to North America and the Europeans who settled on the continent in the early centuries learnt about them from the natives. These herbs, which include the Echinacea and the lobelia inflate, have since gained popularity in Europe.

There are several other herbs valued in North America for their medicinal value, but they were neither local nor adopted from Europe. These ones were introduced to the continent by people from regions in the remaining continents. Among the herb species of foreign origin are the Urtica dioica, commonly known as the stinging nettle, and the Tanacetum vulgare, commonly known as tansy.

BOOK 4

NATIVE AMERICAN

HERBAL RECIPES

CHAPTER 1

EQUIPMENT NEEDED TO EXTRACT & PROCESS HERBS

In order for medicinal herbs to be processed in a way so they will retain their potency and be of maximum use, it is important to use appropriate equipment to pick or extract the material required. Having the suitable tools helps to complete the job quicker and more efficiently.

Tools for Efficient Herb Processing

The reason tool efficiency, particularly with regard to cutting of leaves and branches, is crucial, emanates from the fact that good tools help you make clean cuts. With regard to digging out roots, suitable tools aid you in operating with precision. Hence, you eliminate or minimize damage to the herb, and you end up with minimal losses, if any.

At the same time, using appropriate tools reduces the risk of accidents, such as cuts or bruises, in the course of work. Also, using the right equipment leaves the plant habitat intact and not damaged.

You will now learn the tools you need; that is after you have correctly identified your target herb. This sequence of events is important in order to conduct your wildcrafting appropriately.

You need clippers, knives, saws, trowels and a folding shovel in order to harvest your natural herbs correctly and safely.

Clippers, Scissors & knife

When you have a good quality pair of clippers or scissors, or even knife, the cuts you make when harvesting your herbs are clean, and you do not struggle harvesting even those herbs that are tough, such as Echinacea.

You also have little chance, if any, of hurting your hands or arms in the course of herb harvesting.

The knife has its special role in that it can cut a branch at an angle of 45°, which neither a pair of scissors nor a pair of clippers can manage.

Gloves, paper bags, linen sheets

It is important to wear gloves when harvesting herbs because they protect you from being stung by plants like the stinging nettle; and from being pierced by thorns. The gloves should be the appropriate type to ensure full protection.

Trowel, Folding Shovel & Saw

The trowel and the folding shovel are very useful if you are harvesting roots. This is because there is sometimes plenty of soil you need to dig out. While the trowel would be sufficient for roots that require shallow digging, you need a folding shovel to remove the soil in situations where the roots run deep.

Though big in size, the folding shovel is convenient to carry around because it occupies less space when folded. It is also important to know that shovels are available in varying sizes and also costs; so you can buy as per your needs.

As for saws, they come in handy when you want to harvest herb branches. The reason is that a saw can cut through the thickness of a branch with relative ease, making a clean cut every time. Thus, you minimize the risk of trees becoming infected and being suspected to disease.

Paper Bag & Linen Sheets

It is advisable to note the importance of using linen sheets that are clean at every stage of harvesting herbs. These sheets that are used for storing the herbs once harvested are used all the way from the point of picking the herb to storing the herb at home. In case you cannot find a linen sheet like those traditionally used by Native Americans, it is safe to use a brown paper bag.

Best Herb Harvesting Technique

Normally you become familiar with the best tools for harvesting as you gain herb harvesting experience. This is because you get to learn the tools you need in particular environments, the kind of plants you want, and the specific spots individual plants are located.

There are certain steps you need to take as a beginner, to help you in your journey to becoming a skilled herb harvester. These steps include observing, taking notes, maintaining a sketchbook, and taking photographs.

Becoming Observant

You need to be keen when going around natural habitat with herbs, so you are able to note the different plants in existence, what they look like and how they smell. You also need to register each of the plant's feel to the touch.

Once you get into the habit of observing plants with focus, you get to identify new features and characteristics even in plants considered ordinary. In due course, you will get to learn how individual plants behave during specific seasons, and for some plants how they behave during different years of their life.

Taking Notes

The crucial points you need to write down for personal reference include any plant you have identified, the specific area you found it, the other plants in the vicinity, and any insects in that particular area.

The importance of noting down these factors is that they help you understand the herb growing pattern in the area; hence it becomes easy for you to locate a specific herb without spending too much time.

Maintaining a Sketchbook

Even without special skills in fine art, it is possible to draw a sketch of a plant. At the same time, as long as you understand you are going to sketch the plant, you will, inevitably, be keen in observing it.

As part of your notes, it is advisable to stick some sample flowers and leaves, as well as buds, in your notebook. However, you need to first dry them by placing them in between pages somewhere in the middle of your book.

Taking Photographs

Photographs are great reminders of the plants you are interested in, or those available in the location of your interest. In modern day, cell phones have made this task very easy; you can snap pictures of plants as you move and write down key notes on every one of them.

Rules to Follow for Safe Herb Harvesting

It is very important that certain herb harvesting rules are adhered to, for the purpose of ensuring the herbs you pick are safe for use. After following the recommended rules for some time, you will gain confidence in knowing what herb is good for harvesting and which ones should be given a wide berth.

Identify the Herb First

It is very important that you identify the exact plant you want for your use, keeping in mind there are several plants that are poisonous, yet they look similar to some plants that are edible.

When in doubt, skip harvesting

Any time you are not certain you are looking at the herb you need, avoid harvesting. You had better err on the side of safety; otherwise harvesting a poisonous herb can be fatal.

You should take warning against tasting an herb to check if it tastes the way you expect your target herb to taste. This is a pertinent warning considering there are many plants that look alike; and while some are safe to use, others are dangerous.

Another important reason you need to identify herbs properly and only harvest when you are certain of its identity, is that some plants are among the endangered species in that specific area.

Adhere to the rule of 10%

The rule of 10% holds that when you are on a mission to harvest herbs, for any particular species you find in an area, harvest only 10% of it or less. When you keep to this rule, you help not only to safeguard that particular species, but also to maintain a healthy environment. Overharvesting of herbs can cause fast depletion of natural resources, and hence cause damage to the environment.

Avoid Harvesting in Urban Setups

As a rule, herb harvesting should not be done within or around urban centers. Similarly, it should not be done along roads or railways. Such herbs are normally scanty, and they help to keep the environment healthier than otherwise. Hence there is good reason to spare them.

Be Cautious of Allergies

Since it is unlikely you have used every herb available in the environment, you are certainly not sure how you should respond to some of them. It is, therefore, advisable that you begin by trying out a tiny quantity of a new herb first to rule out the potential for allergic reaction; that is before you can proceed to use the herb for medicinal or culinary use.

Also at the time of testing herbs to ensure you do not react badly to them, caution is given that you only test a single herb at once. This way, if your body responds badly you will be certain of which herb you are allergic to.

Be Vigilant During Harvesting

It is important to be alert and observant all through the herb harvesting mission. This is because, much as you may consider the process an adventure, several dangers lurk within the woods. You could trip on crawling plants, fall into a ditch, be pierced by thorns, be stung by plants like the stinging nettle; and such other forms of harm.

Leave Herbs Alone if their Sap is White

It should be your principle not to harvest any herb that has white sap because most of those herbs have been found to be toxic; and hence, dangerous to use.

Be Keen if the Flowers are in an Umbel

The reason you need to check with keenness any herb whose flowers develop in umbels is that while there are many herbs with healing properties whose flowers develop in this manner, but there are also several dangerous look-alikes.

A good example of a healing herb whose flowers develop in umbels is the yarrow, an herb used to treat depression and generally enhance the health of the brain.

Be Cautious with Herbs like Mushrooms

Much as mushrooms are great herbs hailed for their anti-oxidant properties, you need to check keenly the type you are harvesting. This is because some mushroom species are highly toxic and can cause death.

Herbs from the mint family also need to be checked carefully. There are certain plants that seem to belong to the same family, yet their taste and smells are different. These and other plants that look alike need to be screened before harvesting, to ensure you pick only those you need and which are safe for use. Some among the lookalikes could be poisonous.

It is also important that you do not assume a plant is safe for consumption just because some animal is eating it. Sometimes an animal could consume a dangerous plant without appearing to be harmed, only because that animal has developed tolerance to the poison in that particular plant.

Use of Technology to Identify Plants

Today there are some applications that can help you identify plants, even those you have never seen before. This is in addition to various websites that show images of actual plants and their names.

List of Free Herb Identification Apps

ID Weeds

ID Weeds is an application that the University of Missouri designed, to help in plant recognition. All you are required to do is input certain attributes of the herb you are interested in identifying. The application also has a database of plant pictures that can be of help.

Like That Garden

This application helps when you upload an actual picture of the plant in which you are interested. Once you do this, the application instantly produces the identity of that plant. It should be noted that there is room for error when using this application and others. This is because there are several plants that look similar.

In order to enhance accuracy, use a picture of the plant when its flowers have bloomed; if you are seeking to identify a flowering plant.

Vtree

The firm that developed this application is known as Virginia Technologies. This application is helpful when you want to know the identity of the herbs in your area. Of course, the application has to first establish your position as per the GPS.

The kind of identity this application provides is a combination of herb pictures and the description of every plant shown.

About Herbs

This application provides a plant database, where pictures of plants and their descriptions are provided. In addition, information is provided on simple techniques you can use to prepare medications from the plants.

If you choose to use this application to identify a given plant, it is advisable to use it alongside another of the applications already described.

BOOK 5

HOW TO HANDLE AND STORE HERBAL EXTRACT

t is good to learn how best to handle material extracted from herbal plants, because poor handling can result to loss of potency, deterioration of the material, or even food poisoning.

Best Way to Dry & Store Herbal Preparations

It needs to be remembered that herbal medicine can be extracted from different parts of the plant. For some plants it is the leaves that are medicinal, others the flowers, others the stem, others the roots and the like; while others it is a combination of different parts.

The important point to remember is that there is the preferred way of handling and storing every one of those parts. How best to do the handling and storage depends on which part you are dealing with.

How to handle and dry Plant Bulbs

You should not wash your bulbs after harvest, either to remove dust, insects or such other unwanted items. Instead, you should make a point of shaking off the dirt and any foreign items on the bulbs. If necessary, you can proceed to spread the bulbs along a wall so they can dry very slowly.

How to handle and Dry Tree Stems

If the quantities are suitable, ensure its bundles are attached at the base, making sure also that the bundle diameters are an inch and a half or even less. These, too, can be spread along a wall to dry in a gradual manner.

The best way to handle Plant Barks

Before the bark can be left to dry, it needs to have its exterior peeled off; unless the particular bark needs to be left intact. This process of peeling off the exterior of a bark before drying and storage is referred to as flipping.

The best way to handle Herb Roots

Roots need to be either stretched out or arranged in a circular form. Since any dirt on the roots may not be removed by ordinary rinsing, it may be necessary to use some pressure hose. If the roots are covered in clay, it may even be necessary to brush them off by hand.

For quick and effective drying of roots, it is advisable to slice them lengthwise, especially if they are long or heavy. Note that such splitting of roots is only advisable if they are not aromatic; otherwise their aroma would be lost or marred.

Special Herb Storage Measures

For best storage, you need to ensure the heat the herbs are exposed to is not excessive. The reason is that too much heat can damage the aroma of these herbs, as well as other important components.

Alternatively, in order to retain the potency level of the herbs for the duration of storage when they are exposed to excessive heat, you need to store the herbs in plastic bags of the food-grade type; or even in fiber barrels. If those are not available, you can store your herbs in different containers as long as they are the kind of containers known for emitting oxygen and even moisture.

It is important that every stored herb is labeled, ensuring their source is indicated alongside their date of harvest.

One needs to realize that herbs can easily lose their potency if they are broken or crushed. In short, herbs can retain their potency, and hence their worth, longer when they are stored whole.

Important Herb Growing & Storage Tips

In case you are not relying on wild herbs for your needs but you are, instead, planting your own, there are things you need to know.

First of all, choose to plant herbs that are suitable for your climate. Some plants will not do well in certain environments owing to unfavorable climatic conditions.

In case you want to use seeds to propagate your herbs, as opposed to cuttings or other forms, the common method is to put your seeds inside some container that has water. Such seeds normally sink in and germinate.

Use of pots made of glass or those that are broken for herb growing is discouraged. Another useful tip for growing herbs is that too much watering the plants is bad for the plant and not helpful. It should be done only when the soil has become dry. Excessive watering is not good for herbs.

Once you have harvested your herbs, you can secure them in their fresh form inside a jug with clean water. The parts best stored in such a manner are the plant stems and its leaves.

BOOK 6

BEST NATIVE AMERICAN HERBAL RECIPE

Herb preparations can take different forms, depending on a person's preference, the ailment being treated, and such other factors. The most popular forms of herbal preparations include teas, decoctions, infusions, and ointments.

Recipes for Commonest Herbal Teas

Among the most common herbal teas are raspberry tea, basil tea, mint tea, and such others.

Raspberry, Basil, Mint & Other Popular Teas

Preparation of Raspberry Tea

Ingredients Required

1. Clean water – 8¼ cups

2. Sugar – $^2/_3$ cup

3. Tea bags – 5 packets

4. Raspberry (either fresh or even frozen; also not sweetened) – 4 cups

Method of Preparation

(A)

➢ Pour 4 cupfuls of water in a pan and boil it.

➢ Add the sugar and stir until it dissolves

➢ Next, set the pan aside and drop in the bags of tea.

➢ Steep the mixture for around 7 minutes and then remove the tea bags.

➢ Next, add another 4 cupfuls of water.

(B)

➢ In a different pan, pour in the remainder of the water

➢ Add in the raspberries and put the pan on fire until the mixture boils

➢ Minimize the heat and let the mixture simmer while uncovered

➢ After 3 minutes, strain the mixture and then discard the pulp

➢ Take the raspberry juice produced and mix it with the mixture of tea. Your raspberry tea is now ready for consumption.

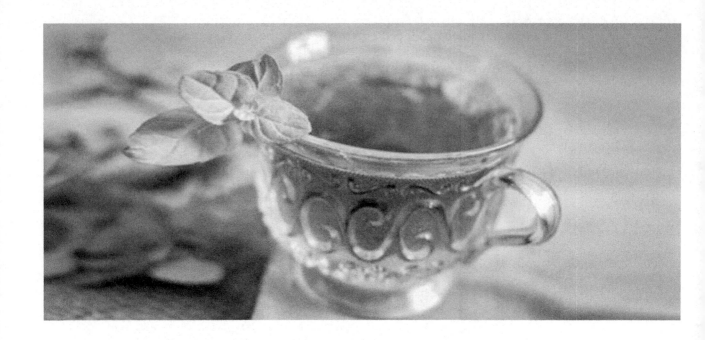

PREPARATION OF BASIL TEA

INGREDIENTS

Required

1. Basil leaves (fresh & finely diced) – 2 tablespoonfuls
2. Hot boiled water – 1 cup

Optional

a. Lemon juice – 3 drops
b. Honey – just enough to taste
c. Ginger (fresh & grated) – 1/3 teaspoonful

METHOD OF PREPARATION

➢ Put the basil & ginger in a tiny pan
➢ Add in the hot boiled water
➢ Leave the mixture to steep and wait 5 minutes
➢ Next, strain the liquid using a fine filter or sieve.
➢ Finally, add your lemon and/or honey if you choose to.

Your basil tea is now ready to drink.

Preparation of Mint Tea

Mint leaves are popular for giving your tea an aroma that is alluring and a flavor that is delicious to the taste. The drink you make using mint leaves is usually referred to as herbal tea, but sometimes it is referred to as tisane.

There are different kinds of mint, and you can use any as you like. For example, sometimes you can use spearmint and other times you can use peppermint for your tea. Of course, there are other herbs in the mint family that you can use for herbal tea.

It is important to note that it is all right to use leaves from different mint plants to make herbal tea. You can, for example, mix spearmint and peppermint for your tea, especially when these herbs are still fresh. It has also been noted that fresh mint leaves have stronger flavor than dried ones.

Whenever you make mint tea, it is advisable to drink it hot; otherwise just drink it ice-cold. You also have the choice to either sweeten the tea or leave it unsweetened. Mint tea is also good with lemon, but it is still fine without the addition; this is as far as taste and potency are concerned.

Ingredients Required

1. Water (after filtration) – 2 cupfuls
2. Peppermint leaves (fresh) – 15

Optional ingredients

a. Honey - 2 teaspoonfuls
b. Slices of lemon – 2
c. Lemon juice – ½ cup
d. Ice – 1 cupful

Method of Preparation

➢ Boil the water

➢ Next, set the boiled water aside and throw in the peppermint leaves

➢ Steep the mixture for 4 minutes or slightly longer, depending on how strong you want your drink to be

> Add in the honey if you so wish.

Your mint tea is ready to drink, but if you wish to garnish it you can use the slices of lemon for that. You can also add lemon juice to modify the taste.

Note:

The above peppermint recipe can be used with any of the other edible mints; like the pineapple, lavender, orange, ginger and the apple mints. It can also be used with the catmint, the calamint, the chocolate mint, and others like the red raripila and licorice mints. Also note that apple mint is the same as woolly mint.

Preparation of Pineapple Mint Tea

Ingredients Required

1. Water – 10 cupfuls

2. Sugar – ½ cup

3. Mint sprigs (fresh) – 8 big ones

4. Tea bags (black) – 8

5. Pineapple juice – 3 cupfuls

6. Lemonade concentrate – 1 can (or 6 ounces)

7. Lemon slices – 3 or more (to serve with)

Method of Preparation

> Put the water in a pan of medium size and let it boil

> Set aside the boiling water and pour in the ½ cup of sugar

> Stir the mixture until the sugar dissolves

> Next put in the black tea bags and cover the pan

> Let the mixture steep for around half an hour

> Next remove the used tea bags

> Pour the tea into a big pitcher

> Add in your pineapple juice and also the lemon concentrate.

You almost have your pineapple mint tea ready; but you need to refrigerate it first. The duration of refrigeration can be as short as one hour, or as long as two full days.

Whatever duration you choose for refrigeration, just remember to retrieve the mint sprigs before you can pour the drink into a pitcher.

Serving of this herbal tea is best done over ice, and alongside your slices of lemon.

GINGER/HIBISCUS TEA

Ginger/Hibiscus tea is the product you get when you prepare herbal tea from the ginger and hibiscus herbs. This natural tea has become very popular over the years, especially because lovers of natural treatments have discovered the potential it has in the process of healing serious ailments.

For instance, the ginger/hibiscus tea has been found to enhance a person's health during the process of chemotherapy. For patients undergoing chemo, this tea has capacity to neutralize the foul taste the medication normally leaves within the mouth.

Ginger/hibiscus tea is also credited with lowering the level of blood pressure, for people whose blood pressure is abnormally high.

It is also good to note that this tea is also delicious and enjoyable to drink; and it is best served over some ice. At the same time, owing to the presence of ginger, the tea is great for enhancing digestion.

The color of the ginger/hibiscus tea is ordinarily a reddish-ruby. As for its potency, it lies in its richness in beta-carotene, flavonoids with anti-oxidant properties, and Vitamin C.

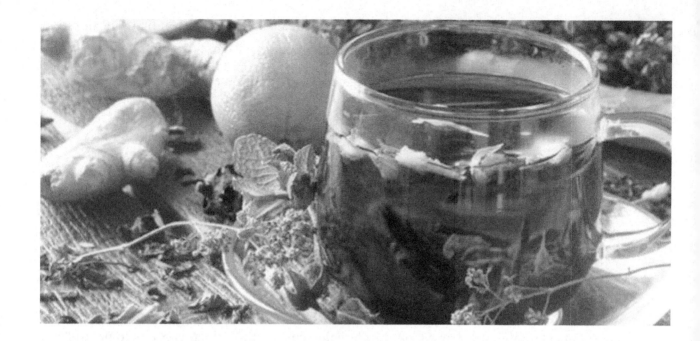

PREPARATION OF GINGER/HIBISCUS TEA

INGREDIENTS REQUIRED

1. Hibiscus flowers (dried) – ¼ cup
2. Ginger (thinly cut) – 2 inches
3. Honey – 1 tablespoon
4. Hot water (boiled) – 7 cups

METHOD OF PREPARATION

➤ Put the hibiscus and the ginger in a pot

➤ Add into the pot the hot boiled water

➤ Leave the mixture to steep for around 5min; if you want the tea stronger, steep for more minutes

➤ Strain your mixture into another container, such as a jug. The liquid you have should be darkish-red in color.

➤ Finally, add in the honey and stir.

Your herbal tea is now ready to drink; and you can serve it either hot or with ice.

How to Make Herbal Decoctions

It is important to note that usually decoctions are made where the part of the herb being used is tough; like when you use the bark, woody stem, or root of the plant. Making a decoction differs from preparing an infusion as the plant parts ordinarily used for infusions include the flowers and leaves, as well as fragile stems.

Decoctions based on Licorice, Burdock & Other Herbs

It is actually not wrong to view decoctions as merely herbal teas with greater concentration than normal.

Preparation of a Licorice Decoction

Ingredients Required

1. Licorice root (dried) – 1 teaspoon
2. Water – 1 cup

Optional ingredient

a. Honey
b. Stevia

Method of Preparation

➢ Pour the water in a heavy pan and heat until it boils
➢ Add in the licorice root and reduce the heat
➢ Let the mixture simmer for around 20 min.
➢ Remove pan from the fire and sieve the mixture.

If you wish to sweeten your decoction a bit, add some honey or even stevia and stir.

NB:

Normally, a decoction is best consumed in amounts ranging from a quarter to a half cup; but sometimes you may vary that amount depending on the type of herb involved.

Preparation of a Burdock Decoction

Ingredients Required

1. Burdock root (fresh) – 2 teaspoons
2. Water – 1 cup

Optional ingredient

a. Honey
b. Stevia

Method of Preparation

➤ Pour the water in a heavy pot and heat up to boiling point

➤ Add in the burdock root and then lower the fire

➤ Leave the mixture to simmer for around 15 min.

➤ Remove the pot from the fire and then sieve your mixture.

You can proceed to add some honey or some stevia if you want to flavor the decoction and to have some sweetness.

Generally, the method of preparing decoctions is the same for most herbs. One of the few variations, nevertheless, comes when you want to either sweeten your decoction or to leave it with its natural flavor.

Another variation is the use of fresh versus dried herbs. For the dried herbs, the ratio of herb to water is 1 teaspoonful to 1 cupful; while for fresh herbs, the ratio is 2 teaspoonfuls to one cupful.

There are several other recipes you can use to prepare herbal decoctions, and you can use the same method as above.

All you need to do is to use different herbs in place of either licorice or burdock. Another herb that produces medicinal herbal decoctions include the yellow dock root, which is effective in the treatment of anemia; and which also has moderate laxative properties.

Other herbs that make great decoctions include the dandelion root that effectively cleanses the liver; the ginseng root, which is effective in hormonal balancing and fighting against fatigue; cinnamon, which is enhances the digestive function, warms the body and fights colds; chicory root, which is great at improving the health of the skin; and the bark of the slippery elm that is used to treat ulcers, diarrhea and also coughs.

How to Make Solar Infusions

Although the technique used in the preparation of herbal teas and infusions is almost similar, it is important to note that the plant material needed for preparation of herbal tea is significantly less than the amount needed to prepare herbal infusion.

At the same time, the time required to steep plant material in the preparation of herbal tea is much less than the time needed for the same when preparing herbal infusions.

One great advantage of having herbal infusions is that they are a great way of preserving the healing properties of herbs. Infusions usually produce herbal oils that have capacity to extend the herbs' shelf-life; meaning the infusions will still be potent and helpful a long time to come.

There is yet another advantage herbal infusions have compared to herbal teas; and that is their potency; infusions are more potent than teas. In case you want to prepare treatment for external use, as in salves and lip balms, an herb infusion serves as a stable base.

The Best Solar Infusion Techniques

When you want to make infusions, the method you need to follow is similar to the one followed when producing tinctures; the major difference being that you use oil as your base in making infusions, but use alcohol when producing tinctures.

The sun's warmth accelerates the infusion making process, while the sun's energy aids in extracting the potent elements from the plant. The sun's role is critical where the plants useful parts cannot be effectively obtained solely through the heating process.

For best herbal infusions, it is advisable to use pure oils from plants; good examples being sunflower oil, almond oil, olive oil and coconut oil. Many people prefer to use olive oil in their herb infusion process because it can safely last longer at normal room temperature.

During the infusion process, the ratio of herb to oil is not fixed. A lot is left to your preference and how potent you want your infusion to be. Nevertheless, when new to herbal infusions, it is advisable to start off your ratio of dry herbs to oil at 1 to 10 ounces.

Preparation of a Solar Infusion – Rosemary

It is best to use olive oil when making a solar herb infusion because of the oil's long shelf-life.

Ingredients required

    a. Rosemary (dried) – 1 ounce

    b. Olive oil – 10 ounces

Method of Preparation

1. Take your dried rosemary and chop it finely. If you choose to wash the herbs first, wait until they have dried completely before use. This is because your herbal infusion can easily get spoilt if the herb has excessive water in it.

2. Put the fine herb material in a glass jar

3. Add in the oil and stir to mix the contents

4. Next, put the lid on and label that container with a name and date. This is important especially if you are making other herbal infusions; it is easy to confuse the herbs once they have been chopped.

5. Put your jar next to a window where sunshine can reach; although you have a choice to place it at a different location as long as that place is warm.

6. Leave the jar contents to rest for around 2½ weeks.

7. Make a point of stirring the contents once everyday; and as you do so push the herb material beneath the olive oil.

8. If there is some condensation on the underside of the jar lid, wipe it off. Do the same for any condensation you may find above the surface of the oil. It is crucial to do this clearance in order to prevent the herbal infusion from having excess moisture. The danger with the moisture content being too high in the herbal infusion is that there is the risk of the infusion developing mold.

9. Finally, sieve mixture and pour the infused oil into a dark colored glass container.

10. Label the container with the infused content and store it in a location that is cool and away from direct sunlight. Storing your herbal infusion under these conditions maximizes its shelf-life.

Oven & Stove-based Oil Infusions

It is possible to prepare herbal oil infusions faster than it takes to make them via using solar. This means you would need to put your herbal mixture directly on fire.

Ingredients required

1. Citrus peelings (fresh) – 2 tablespoons
2. Olive oil – 10 tablespoons

Method of Preparation

➢ Prepare a double boiler by putting a glass jar in a shallow pot of water

➢ Put the citrus peelings in the jar

➢ Add in the oil and mix

➢ Now switch on the fire and let the water heat

➢ Leave the mixture of citrus peelings and oil to simmer at low heat for around 5 hours

➢ Finally, sieve the contents of the glass jar and discard the solids. The liquid is your herbal infusion made through direct heating.

This kind of infusion needs to be stored in a refrigerator; but before you do that it is important that you label the jar in a manner to identify the content, and to show the date of its preparation.

Recipes for Herbal Ointments

Natural ointments are usually gentle to the skin, yet they have capacity to treat scrapes that are often painful, and rashes that are usually itchy. They also enhance the health of dry and dull skin.

Beyond the role of treatment that herbal salves, lotions and other ointments serve, there is also their capacity to enhance absorption of nutrients through the skin.

Salves made from Calendula, Peppermint, Chamomile, Eucalyptus & Other Herbs

How to Make an Herbal Salve

Ingredients Required:

1. Tea tree essential oil – 4 drops

2. Calendula flower petals (fresh) – 2 tablespoons

3. Coconut oil – ½ cup

4. Beeswax – 1 tablespoon

Method of Preparation

➢ Pour the coconut oil in a small container

➢ Add in the tea tree oil

➢ Add in the calendula flower petals and stir to mix

➢ Put water in a pan

➢ Immerse your small jug into the pan and switch on the heat source

➢ Keep the fire on until the water in the pan begins to boil

➢ Reduce the fire level and let the herb mixture continue heating for around 45 minutes.

➢ Pour the herb mixture through some cheese cloth and into a bowl. As the cheesecloth holds the herb remnants, the oil infusion is collected in the bowl.

➢ Make a point of squeezing out the cheese cloth with your hands, so that whatever remaining little infusion remains in the plant remnants can drop into the bowl.

You have just made a double-boiler and used it to make your oil infusion.

- ➢ Next, put the beeswax in a container and melt it
- ➢ Add the liquefied beeswax into the bowl containing the oil infusion and stir to mix
- ➢ Put the mixture into small containers of your choice
- ➢ Store the containers in the refrigerator for around a quarter of an hour

By the end of this period, your mixture should have solidified into the medicinal salve you want.

How to Make Herbal Creams

The same technique explained above, the one used to make an herbal salve, works for an herbal cream with only a little adjustment. This small difference is that you need to use a lesser amount of beeswax when making a cream compared to when you are making a salve.

For instance, in the case where a salve requires a tablespoon of beeswax, a cream would require a teaspoon of this substance.

BOOK 7

HOW TO EXTRACT HERBAL OIL FOR TREATMENT

Herbal oils represent essential oils produced naturally, as opposed to being made in science laboratories. Many of these have medicinal properties, culinary value, or both. The method of oil extraction may vary from one type of plant to another.

You can also consider essential oils as those liquids produced when plant extracts are combined with solvents. They are like parts of the plant preserved in liquefied form.

Among the popular methods of herbal oil extraction is steam distillation and solvent extraction. These two are common in extraction of herbal oil for healing purposes. Nevertheless, there are other effective ways of extracting herbal oils; many of these oils being put into different uses like cooking and skin health. Among these methods is maceration, water distillation and enfleurage, and cold press extraction.

Whichever method you choose to extract your oil needs to be appropriate for the herb involved. This is important for purposes of maintaining the quality and integrity of the oil. Among the important factors to consider when identifying the most suitable technique to use in extracting your herbal oil are the temperature involved as well as the pressure.

To understand why some methods used in extracting herbal oil are considered better than others depending on the type of plant, or even the part of plant involved, consider extraction of oil from the peels of a citrus fruit.

It is more suitable to use cold press for this purpose rather than using enfleurage, for the reason that it is necessary to pierce the peelings and subsequently squeezing them. Obviously, it is more effective to use the extraction method in this case than trying to use enfleurage.

How to use Steam for Oil Distillation

The method of steam distillation is very popular as a method of extracting herbal oils from natural plants. The oils extracted, which are commonly referred to as essential oils, are isolated in the course of this distillation process, and they are normally used as crucial components of some natural products.

The steam distillation method of obtaining herbal oil works as steam drives the relevant plant compounds to vaporize, after which they condense and are subsequently collected.

The Process of Steam Distillation

1. Begin by putting your plant material in a container known as a 'still,' ordinarily made of stainless steel.

2. Inject steam into the container via some inlet, so that the steam effectively covers the plant matter. The contact of steam and plant material causes the release of plant molecules with aromatic and healing properties; and at this stage they are in the form of vapor.

3. Have a condenser or just a condensation flask ready to receive the vaporized compounds. The condenser is made in such a way that one of its pipes facilitates exit of the hot water while the other gives room for entry of the cold water. Once the herbal vapor has entered the condenser, it quickly turns back into a liquid.

4. It is important to have something known as a separator at the bottom of the condenser; the place where the liquid settles after condensation from vapor. This liquid contains not only oil but also water. As would be expected owing to their varying densities, the oil floats on the water, and so you can siphon off the herbal oil with ease.

5. For the few types of herbal oil of greater density than water, like oil from the clove, you will find it beneath the water; and you can pour out the water to remain with the oil.

How to Maintain the Integrity of Herbal Oil

Maintaining integrity of herbal oil starts at harvesting of the plant material, proceeds to cleaning and storage, and continues up to the extraction and processing of the herb material, up to its storage.

It is important that the herb material harvested is inspected and duly sorted as soon as harvesting is done. While still at the site of harvesting, for example, you need to ensure the plant material you have assembled is pure or appropriate. This is the point at which you should get rid of any extraneous matter; like dirt, unwanted crawling insects or other plant material, parts of the herb known to be toxic, bugs, rotten sections of the plant, and even any part of the herb with no medicinal value.

In modern day, it is advisable that people doing the sorting of required plant material wear masks and even gloves for protection against dust, unwanted smells, and such other unfavourable elements.

Herb Processing at Primary Level

It is crucial to ensure primary processing is carried out properly. Processing at primary level entails washing of the raw plants. Roots, tubers and rhizomes need special attention, ensuring they are not only washed with water that is clean, but also well dried soon after.

Soaking of herbs, be it the root or any other part, should be kept at a minimum period unless it is of absolute necessity.

Also, it is important that the water used for cleaning the herb material be changed frequently, to ensure the material is finally clean.

Leaching, which means having water run over the raw plants, can be done if found necessary for effective cleaning of the material. Nevertheless, this process should be limited to the minimum time necessary, in order to prevent unnecessary loss of active content.

Ageing of Herbs

It may be necessary to age some herbs before the actual extraction of medicinal portions, and this involves storage of the material for a specified period. Depending on the particular plant, the herbal material can be aged under direct sunshine or under some shade.

The essence of ageing is to have excessive moisture removed through evaporation; and sometimes for hydrolysis or such other enzymatic reaction to take place. For some herbs, the aging process leads to modification of their chemical make-up.

A good example is aging of the cascara bark. Once the bark of the cascara plant has been aged for a year or longer, its components that have irritating effect are rendered non-consequential. For that reason, the herb material can be used for its therapeutic value without fear of the irritating side effects.

Cascara is known to treat constipation as it has laxative properties, and it is also effective in the treatment of gallstones.

Herb Sweating

Some herbs require sweating, a process that involves oxidizing and even hydrolysing some of the herbs' chemical components. A good example of herb sweating is the process of fermentation.

Under this process, the plant material is kept under temperatures between 45° to 65° centigrade; and under very humid conditions. Depending on which herb is involved, fermentation can take a week or as long as 2 whole months.

A good example of herb sweating is the sweating of vanilla beans. These ones are laid densely together between thick blankets, like those made of wool, and then exposed to sunlight in the day. In the night, these well packed vanilla beans are put into boxes that are properly covered with woollen material. This process goes on repeatedly for a period of around 2 months.

By the end of this period, the vanilla beans are expected to have significantly lost weight – ordinarily around 80% of it. They will also have acquired their unique color and scent.

Herb Blanching

Herb blanching, also referred to as herb parboiling, requires that you put the herbs in boiling water after you have washed them; and let them boil for a short while. The idea is to remove the herbs before they can get fully cooked.

This process serves a variety of purposes; one being improvement of the herb's shelf-life, following the gelatinization of the plant starch. Others involve preventing mould from developing, and insects from contaminating the plant matter.

Blanching of herbs also hastens their drying. For other herbs like the almond, blanching makes it easy to process them, because the coating of the seeds is effectively removed.

Herb Steaming/Boiling

This process of boiling or even steaming herbs entails cooking them in some liquid like water or even vinegar; or even milk or wine.

As steaming takes place, the plant matter is separated from the water that is boiling, but the steam reaches it directly. This results in the texture of the plant material becoming moist.

Usually, the plant material is put into a steamer, while in other instances the plant material is pre-mixed with wine, vinegar or even brine prior to the steaming process. In case you do not have access to a steamer, you can use a unique utensil set with some sort of flat frame, and which you can suspend over some water that is boiling.

One of the important roles steaming plays is softening of the herb tissue, so the enzymes in the matter are denatured. Another role this process plays is thermally degrading targeted chemical components.

There are also times when an excipient is used, and it ends up being absorbed into the herb tissue. A good example is when the root of the moldenke herb is steamed alongside the black bean. For those who like taking the moldenke decoction as a tonic, they find its effect more enhanced when the herb is steamed together with the black bean.

Herb Baking/Roasting

By baking or even roasting herb material, you end up drying the matter using indirect heat or what is termed diffused heat. This process is often referred to as dry heating. All you need to do is put your plant material in some kind of heating source.

Often, people who use the baking or roasting technique embed their plant material in some talc powder, or what is essentially magnesium silicate. The reasoning behind this covering is that the material can be heated at high temperatures, but have the heat evenly distributed over the surface of the herb material.

To further enhance the efficacy in even heat distribution, some people wrap the plant material in some moistened paper; and it remains this way for the entire process of herb roasting. Good examples of herbs that need to be roasted before they can be used for their healing properties include the nutmeg and the kudzu.

While the nutmeg herb is known for its strong anti-oxidant properties, regulation of blood pressure and such other health benefits, the kudzu herb is renowned for its capacity to fight dependence on alcohol, metabolic issues and such other health properties.

Herb Stir-Frying

By stir-frying is meant the process of putting plant material into some frying pan or even a pot that is being heated; and continuing to stir or toss the material for some time. The aim is to continue this process until the plant material changes its outer color to look charred; or the look of having been carbonized.

Sometimes stir-frying may need some wine or vinegar to act as adjuvant; or even honey, ginger juice or saline. Any of these adjuvants can be easily infused into the plant environment, so it becomes part and parcel of the plant material in its processed form.

It is recommended that sand, clay, bran, or such other appropriate material be admixed with the plant material to ensure even distribution of heat over the exterior of the plant material.

A good example of admixing herbal material with suitable substances for the sake of even heating is the case of the liquorice root and honey. Other suitable examples of admixing while stir-frying involve mixing the bunge root with wine, and ginger with sand. In the case of ginger, it is stir-fried alongside the sand to a point where the ginger's surface changes to brown.

BOOK 8

BEST FLOWER-BASED REMEDIES

There are many plant flowers whose value is not only aesthetic but is also medicinal. Some of them treat cognition-related issues, such as dyslexia, memory loss and even stuttering; while others treat physical illnesses like hypertension, allergies and asthma, migraines, and others that arise from psychological problems.

Among the commonest flower remedies is aromatherapy, which is primarily based on the nice smelling flowers.

Another is skin care, which is based on natural oils as well as ointments extracted from the flowers.

Another common flower remedy is enhancement of body metabolism, which is based on the teas and the infusions made from various plant flowers.

There is also the self-care remedy that is based on the essences of different flowers depending on the person's need. It should be noted that for every therapeutic flower, there is the spiritual need it serves; and this becomes the bases for different cures, especially of a psychological nature.

Another popular flower remedy is treatment of insomnia. This remedy involves preparation of flower satchels, which are basically packets of fragrant flowers. You are supposed to put these in strategic places where you frequent, and particularly under your pillow for enhancement of quality sleep.

Damiana-Turnera Diffusa, Mullein-Verbascum & Others

While the yellow flowers of the damiana plant, also known as the turnera diffusa, are used as aphrodisiacs just like the plant leaves, those tiny yellow ones of the mullein-verbascum are used as treatment for serious coughs such as whooping cough and tuberculosis.

Jasmine Flower Healing

Jasmine flowers are used for mood improvement and treatment of depression. Its healing efficacy emanates from the capacity of the flower extracts to regulate breathing while also regulating blood pressure.

The oil extracted from these flowers also soothes tough muscles and rejuvenates the body, helping to eliminate aches in different parts of the body and even helps cramps.

Extracts from jasmine flowers have additional health benefits, including enhancement of the digestive function and management of ulcers.

Calendula Flower Healing

The petals of the calendula flowers are credited with successful treatment of cuts and burns; and all wounds in general.

The flowers have anti-bacterial as well as anti-inflammatory properties, and for this reason they are effective in the treatment of skin rashes and acne, as well as athlete's foot. The ointments, creams and oils produced from the calendula flowers are popular because their ingredients are pure; hence effective.

The calendula flowers have also been found to be helpful in easing menstrual pain as well as muscle spasms. Since the calendula herb is also a potent astringent, its flower extracts are effective in eliminating harmful bacteria from inside the mouth. As a result, their products are used for maintenance of oral health.

Healing Power of Lavender

Flowers of the lavender plant are used to help the person relax, and to rejuvenate both the body and the mind. People who develop such high level of anxiety that they have problems sleeping can rely on medicine from lavender flowers for treatment.

Also, owing to the anti-inflammatory and also antiseptic properties of oil extracted from lavender flowers, it is used in the treatment of burns and general wounds, as well as alleviation of acne.

The Healing Properties of the Rose

Rose flowers are not only mood lifting when gifted in form of a bouquet, but also when used as herbal medication. Rose herbal treatment enhances blood circulation and fights anxiety as well as depression. It is thus a deterrent to heart-related ailments and stroke.

The healing effect of the rose flower is made stronger by the flower's anti-oxidant properties, which are a result of its richness in Vitamin C. Rose flowers are also credited with relief of infections and capacity to fight viruses.

The Healing Properties of the Passion Flower

The passion flower has for many years been used as a sedative. In modern day, this flower has been found to have additional medicinal value, which includes treatment of stress and anxiety, as well as insomnia and panic. The medication made from the passion flower is also effective in the treatment of depression.

Delicious Honey with Healing Properties

70% to 80% of honey is sugar, but this popular bee product also contains minerals, protein and a proportion of water. This means it is nutritious to the body. As for treatment, honey is known as a great solution for allergies and the sore throat; but it also treats several other ailments.

Some of the illnesses honey treats include bacterial infections and unnecessary drying of wounds. The viscosity of honey is responsible for providing a protective layer to wounds and hindering infection.

For the treatment of burns, salves are prepared from honey; and it is credited with hastening the burns' duration of healing. It has been found that it takes a shorter time for honey to make a wound sterile than it takes other medications. Besides, the healing of honey ensures the scar from the wound is minimal.

Honey is also credited with memory enhancement; and this is particularly so for women of menopausal or even post-menopausal age. In fact, research conducted on honey treatment established that women who consumed tualang honey for a number of weeks had their memory improve just as well as those put on hormone-based estrogen plus progestin therapy.

Some other research has found that honey is effective in the treatment of herpes; both oral and even genital. Honey is also great at healing lesions caused by herpes just like ointments sold in pharmacies. In fact, honey has been found to reduce itchiness from such lesions more effectively.

Honey is also credited with controlling diabetes, and this is from the fact that the glycemic index of honey is lower than that of sugar. In essence, therefore, although honey is sweet, it does not spike the sugar level in the blood. Researchers have found that people who replace their use of sugar with consumption of honey manage to maintain steady and healthy levels of blood sugar.

Also, some research has indicated that owing to its anti-oxidant properties honey has capacity to mitigate multiplication of cancer cells. On that basis, these researchers who conducted their study in 2011 recommended further research be done on the potential of honey to effectively treat cancer.

Honey is also credited with boosting immunity, which means it helps the body to ward off disease. It also has anti-microbial properties, which result from its capacity to carry out enzymatic generation of hydrogen peroxide.

However, there is another variety of honey known as manuka, and though it has no peroxide, it is still rich in anti-bacterial properties. It is important to understand that a major reason honey prevents microbes from multiplying is its low level of pH coupled with its high concentration of sugar.

Honey specifically made for medical purposes is rich in anti-bacterial properties; and it is a particularly strong antibiotic against those bacteria resistant to other medications. Honey comes in handy especially because bacteria that are resistant to medications end up becoming a threat to life.

It is important to note that the richness of honey with regard to its anti-microbial properties depends greatly on where its nectar originated from.

Best Herbal Syrups & Tinctures

The distinction between syrup and a tincture is that the thick fluid that is the syrup contains a high level of sugar; and other times it is just a liquid with viscous. In the meantime, a tincture gives color or pigmentation to material; or it dyes it.

There are several plant-based syrups with healing properties, and many have come with the benefit of settling well in drinks and even desserts. In addition to introducing healing potential to the drinks, such syrups also add flavor to those particular drinks.

In fact, there are as many ways of consuming healing syrups as your creativity can allow; meaning you can create your own recipe into which to incorporate some healing syrup. All you need to do is learn the basics of preparing herbal syrup and you can adopt it but use your preferred herbal syrup.

One caution, though, is that you need to establish if the particular herbal syrup has any contraindication, and if any, what the limitations of consuming that particular herbal product are.

How to Prepare Herbal Syrup

It is important that you decide in advance the sweetening method you want to follow when preparing your syrup. The major methods for sweetening herbal syrup are use of sugar or even honey; and the longevity of the syrup is mainly dependent on the substance used to sweeten it.

Difference in Longevity of Syrup

When honey is used as the sweetener, the shelf-life of the syrup normally around 3mths; but when the sweetening substance is sugar the shelf-life of the syrup can be as long as 6mths.

The reason for this variation is that sugar has better capacity of locking in sugar than any honey has; essentially meaning that sugar-based syrup has less water. It is crucial to understand that water is paramount in the development of mold and bacteria. It, therefore, takes longer for sugar-based syrup to go bad than the one based on honey.

Nevertheless, irrespective of the kind of sweetener used, you need to store your syrup in a refrigerator as a precautionary measure.

Another measure you can take to enhance longevity of your syrup is to add some alcohol to it during preparation; ordinary added in form of an alcohol-based herbal infusion. If you decide to add an alcohol herbal infusion, ensure it occupies a quarter of your syrup bottle.

You need to keep in mind that it is an option for people to add or not to add alcohol or alcohol-based tinctures to their syrups. Hence there is no standard longevity duration for home-made syrups. For that reason, you need to observe your home-made syrup very well beforehand to make sure it is still fit for consumption.

How to Tell if Syrup is Stale

Some of the obvious signs herbal syrup is stale or unfit to consume include having visible growth or some odd smell. Experts advise that if you have doubts regarding the freshness of any syrup, choose caution and dispose of it.

Effect of Herb Type

You need to give serious consideration to the herb type or types to use in preparing your syrup, as that will determine the healing properties that syrup is going to have.

You also need to consider the best method to follow in preparing your natural concentrate, which you are going to use in preparing your syrup. You can either base your syrup making on a decoction or some concentrated tea.

Basically your method of choice should be determined by the herb you have.

Herbs that Require Decoctions

If you are going to use berries, plant roots or even bark to prepare your concentrate, you need to use the decoction method.

In this method, the ratio of herb to water ought to be 1:1.

In the process of heating your mixture, ensure it simmers on your stove while uncovered until such a time as the amount is halved.

Herbs that Require Concentrated Tea

Among the herb parts requiring use of strong or concentrated tea are flowers and also leaves.

Method of Preparing Herbal Syrup

You need to boil the water first using a pot, and then you add in your herbs. The ratio of water to herbs ought to be 1:1.

After the water is boiled and you have put in your herbs, remove the pot from the heat source and proceed to cover it using some lid. You should leave the herb mixture in that state for around half an hour, to allow for steeping.

To ensure you have extracted the greatest portion of the medicinal part of the herb, it is imperative that you make use of the correct extraction technique.

When to Adjust Ratios

Sometimes you may need to adjust the ratio of herb to water upwards when preparing concentrates, for herbs which happen to be volatile; with the herb portion being greater. Examples of such herbs include peppermint and even cinnamon.

Conversely, you may need to adjust the ratio of herb to water downwards when it comes to herbs that are gentler; often those with little aroma. Examples of such herbs include plantain and even hawthorn.

Once you have completed preparing the concentrate, make a point of measuring your final product. This is important for establishing the exact amount of concentrate at your disposal.

The next step should be to heat that concentrate on low fire, before adding in your sweetener. The ratio of concentrate to sweetener ought to be 1:1.

You need to stir the concentrate mixture up to the point where it becomes sufficiently sticky to layer the back of any spoon. At this point, remove the mixture from the source of heat and let it cool properly.

In the event you plan on using alcohol or alcohol-based tincture, you need to put it in your chosen syrup bottle, and see that it goes quarter-way. The next step is to pour your cool syrup into the same bottle, and to shake the mixture until everything is evenly spread.

The final step involves labeling your syrup bottle. The details should include the name or names of the herbs used, and the exact date you have prepared the syrup.

Note:

It is inappropriate to add alcohol or alcohol-based tincture to the syrup you are preparing before the syrup is completely cooled. The reason is that doing so interferes with the stabilizing capacity of the alcohol.

Syrup Recipe for Stomach Upset

Ingredients Required

1. Ginger root (fresh) – 1 cup

2. Cinnamon – 6 sticks

3. Water – 2 cups

4. Sugar – 1 cup

5. Brandy (optional) – ¼ of the syrup bottle

Note that sugar can be substituted with honey.

Method of Preparation

Use the decoction technique to prepare the herb concentrate for use, when making this herbal syrup.

Ginger/Cinnamon Syrup Health Benefits

The ginger in the syrup helps to clear nausea while stimulating the digestive function.

As for cinnamon, not only does it aid in digestion, but it also helps to eliminate stomach upsets and also discomfort.

Owing to the healing properties of cinnamon, this syrup also contributes to controlling the level of sugar in the blood; meaning it minimizes risks of developing type 2 diabetes.

Caution in Ginger Use

Use ginger and even cinnamon in moderation because consuming great amounts at once can lead to irritation of the mouth, and even the throat.

As for ginger specifically, anyone with ulcers of the stomach should not use it as it could aggravate the situation.

According to the National Center for Complementary and Integrative Health, or NCCIH, there are some risks in taking too much ginger. Christa Brown, who is licensed in California as a dietician and nutritionist, advises individuals to limit consumption of ginger to a maximum of 3 or 4 grams each day.

The reason is that ginger has been found to cause side effects to certain individuals after their day's consumption reached 6g or over. Besides risking irritation of the mouth and the throat, taking too much ginger can cause heartburn, problems of digestion, vulnerability to bleeding, and kidney problems.

In fact, the National Kidney Foundation has listed ginger as an herb you should avoid if you are already on medication; reason being ginger could interfere with the efficacy of that other medication.

Caution in Cinnamon Use

People should also be alert when consuming syrups that contain cinnamon, especially if they are using other medications. This is because cinnamon has blood-thinning effect, and consuming it alongside medications with similar effects can be dangerous.

This particular recipe is most beneficial to anyone suffering indigestion and nausea, or different gastro-intestinal problems.

As for the timing, you can consume syrup that contains cinnamon either before taking meals or following a meal. Either way, it will help in enhancing digestion.

BOOK 9

NATIVE AMERICAN HERBAL DISPENSATORY

CHAPTER 1

SPIRITUALITY & HEALING FOR THE NATIVE AMERICAN

While many Americans and people of the world have embraced herbal medicine as practiced by the natives of their respective countries, many of them do not practice the spiritual aspect of it.

Spirituality, Healing & Relevant Rituals

Spirituality, especially for the Native Americans, played a central role in the healing process. They believed that every object and being in the world has a connection to nature. At the same time, their belief was that spirits exist with power to cause disease and to give good health.

These health matters were not limited to the physical body, according to the Native Americans; they also included emotional health. They also included the harmony one enjoyed not only with the society to which he/she belonged, but also with the environment. Health, therefore, from the perspective of the Native American, is comprehensive; and the health of the society and the environment must also be sought.

For practical purposes, when an individual was ailing, people of his/her community would gather to hold ceremonies; and here they would pray, dance, chant and partake of herbal treatments.

The process of treatment is different today. Many people opt for science based medicine; the modern medicine.

Role of the Traditional Healers

The healers among the Native Americans were referred to as 'shamans' by the Europeans who came and settled in North America. However, the natives would refer to them as medicine men/women or simply healers.

The role played by the healers was mainly obtaining the spiritual world, and in particular the creator or that which they referred to as the 'supreme spirit.' This they did for the purposes of improving the welfare of the person concerned or the community as a whole.

A medicine man was not only a traditional doctor; he was also a priest. As healers, medicine men were well trained in handling ailments of every kind; and the people believed that causes of illnesses are not necessarily natural, but they can also be supernatural.

Healers' Attire & Performance

Traditional healers wore masks that were often ghastly and bizarre; the aim being to scare away the spirit responsible for causing pain or illness.

They would shake rattles and beat drums as they danced around the affected person, for the purposes of exorcising the demons within him/her. This act of exorcism was carried out to complement the use of herbal substances in treating the ailing person. At times, animal products were used as part of the treatment, in addition to other techniques.

Today, healers often use cups or even suction tubes to strengthen a person's healing potential. They also use purification techniques as well as purging; and these procedures are meant to complement the use of herbal treatments.

Inherited Healing Skills

Experts in herbal medicine have often inherited the skills from their forefathers; one generation passing the skills to the next. For some, though, they get into the practice because something inspired them to do so.

For someone to qualify to practice traditional medicine, he/she is required to spend a significant amount of time as a trainee; being taught by a medicine man/woman with great experience.

Tools Medicine Men/Women Used

Medicine men and women were known to use skins and fur shells as tools of trade. They also use roots, feathers, bone and crystals in a similar manner.

As for feathers, they would be used to carry the message meant for the Supreme or Great Spirit; being linked not only to the air, but also to the wind. There are times when the healer would get into a trance, and in while in that state acquire the assistance of spiritual guides.

Traditional Healing Rituals

Native Americans carried out symbolic rituals as part of the treatment process; basically to try and bring peace to the people in attendance, their respective environments, and their tribes as well. Various ceremonies were also done for such purposes.

Ceremonies were meant to bring harmony within groups of people, but not to heal individuals. There were tribes like the Sioux, and even the Navajo, who would make use of medicine wheels, singing, dancing and sacred hoops during rituals. Such rituals would last days, but the exact durations varied from on tribe to another.

Connection of Native American Traditions & Modern Medicine

For many years, the US government was averse to the traditional practices of the Native American, and it sought to suppress them.

Ban on Traditional Practices

Starting 1882, the US federal government decided to ban any religious right Native Americans enjoyed, in an attempt to curb the influence these natives had on methods of treatment.

According to Henry Teller who served as Interior Secretary at the time, the methods of treatment used by the Native Americans hindered civilization. He prohibited further engagements in native ceremonies and the accompanying dances.

This ban was subsequently supported by the Commissioner for Indian Affairs, Hiram Prince, who in 1883 produced a report indicating there was no good reason for Indians to continue engaging in practices that repulsed morality and common decency.

The Native Americans did not take this ban kindly and they ignored it. Sadly, toward the end of 1890, the government, through the 7th Cavalry, killed around a hundred and fifty of them as they participated in one of their traditional dances, although apparently the directive had been to arrest the participants.

Nevertheless, it is worth noting that this particular dance, dubbed 'Ghost Dance,' did not confine itself to matters of personal healing, but also encompassed the administrative welfare of the community. In fact, it is said that among the matters covered in the dance was some prophesy that dominance by the whites would come to an end, albeit in a non-violent manner.

The fact that the dance ceremony encouraged Native Americans to live clean and be honest did not deter the government from discouraging it. The noble idea promoted by the dance, encouraging people to extend a hand of assistance beyond cultural borders was also ignored.

Even though the killing of innocent civilians, including children, was condemned by everyone, the perpetrators were set free after trial. After a period of 2 years, the Commissioner for Indian Affairs, Thomas Morgan, pronounced a jail term of 6 months or thereabouts for any native found to be practicing traditional medicine or engaging in any religious dance. Moving forward, several other steps were taken to suppress the natives' religious habits and practices.

As a consequence, the Native Americans were not able to effectively practice traditional healing beyond 1900. The Indian Health Service or IHS began to establish clinics and modern hospitals at the beginning of the 20th century, from where physical injuries and other illnesses were treated.

This means treatment was provided to the community in these modern facilities, without the spiritual aspect Native Americans so much valued. One of the reasons the natives gave in and sought treatment in these facilities was that people had begun to suffer afflictions formerly alien to them. They termed these 'white-man' diseases; and they did not have any traditional way of treating them.

Redemption of Traditional Healing

The Religious Freedom Act which was passed in 1978 set the Native Americans free to practice their spiritual beliefs, which had traditionally been embedded in the traditional healing practices.

Unfortunately, after so many years of not being allowed to engage in their traditional ceremonies, the healing aspect the natives remembered was devoid of its original richness.

Those who remembered some traditional healing practices preferred to safeguard it within their respective tribes. Even those who are prepared to share it with other Indian tribes are not at ease sharing it with foreigners; people not of Indian descent.

There is some belief among some that sharing traditional healing information with outsiders can potentially weaken the spiritual potency of the medicine.

Practice of Herbal Medicine Today

Today, the American society has accepted that both traditional and modern practice of medicine can work in tandem with each other. With this open mindedness, the traditional healing methods practiced by Native Americans are becoming popular by the day.

In fact, many people have come to believe not only is it important to address people's physical and mental states, but also their spiritual wellbeing. Those who do not practice the spiritual aspect of healing, at least, respect other people's views about it.

After all, there are many people with reservations regarding the potential for pharmaceutical products to be addictive, toxic, or have side effects. Such people are leaning more toward natural healing, a good part of which is borrowed from the practices of the Native American.

It is now generally accepted that several Native American products of great quality have for decades served the people well in addressing different ailments. It is also acknowledged that although the herbal treatments traditionally used do not provide an accurate measure or dosage, they are not as toxic as modern drugs treating the same ailments.

In short, Americans have realized they can substitute pharmaceutical medications for herbal treatments and avoid negative side effects.

The important thing to do if buying herbal remedies is to go through the ingredients listed, so as to note the herbs used. Hence you will be able to see if there is one you have reservations about because of potential personal complications, such as allergies, inappropriateness when pregnant, and interactions with pharmaceuticals you are already using.

In short, just as care is needed before taking any modern medicine, care should be taken before taking any herbal medications.

In summary, herbal treatments by the Native American have been in practice long in history, and they did not begin when American settlers began documenting them. However, these treatments are now on record, and their documentation is being continually improved as an integral segment of alternative treatment.

Native Americans are becoming particularly aware of the value of their traditional treatments, and they are being embraced by other communities. They have noted that many individuals and organizations have taken the same botanicals traditionally used, and processed them into food and other health supplements.

Native Americans relied on over 2,800 herb species, and a good number of those are now in use for the manufacture of modern supplements.

The value of herbal medicines as used by Native Americans has not only been embraced by North Americans; the larger world has acknowledged it. In fact, the market for traditional remedies in form of herbal products has already hit an annual mark of $60 billion.

CHAPTER 2

HERBAL EXTRACTS FOR RADIANCE & HYGIENE

There are several effective and safe herbal products you can use to keep your skin radiant even as you exercise proper hygiene.

One of the ways to maintain a healthy skin, besides feeding on nutritious food, is ensuring the skin is free from disease.

Herbal Extracts for Skin Treatments

Among the ailments notorious for destroying the health of the skin are abscesses, such as boils, and gingivitis. Abscesses usually emerge beneath the skin and swell, and also produce pus. They generally appear as reddish bumps.

Sometimes these bumps are painful, and they continue increasing in size until such a time as someone removes them.

For boils and such other abscesses to develop, bacteria will have invaded the skin and afflicted the hair follicles. Sometimes they expand and acquire the size of baseballs. In addition to developing a reddish color, these boils and their surrounding skin become sore.

Experts advise against picking at such boils, because doing so could cause further infection within the surrounding regions. Alternatively, it could lead the infection deeper into the body as opposed to remaining close to the surface. Such aggravation of infection can also occur if the boil is not properly drained after treatment.

Common Herbal Remedies for Abscesses

Indian Sorrel Treatment

The Indian Sorrel, otherwise called Sarvajjaya, is effective in the treatment of boils and similar abscesses. The potent part of the herb for this purpose comprises the plant leaves, whose extract needs to be applied two times a day on the affected region of the body.

This leaf matter is made into poultice form for the purpose of application.

Alternatively, you can ground the fresh leaves, heat some little water and mix it with the pounded material to form some paste. All you need thereafter is to apply this herbal paste several times a day onto the affected area of the body.

Aloe Vera Treatment

The Aloe Vera plant, otherwise known as Gheekumari, has medicinal leaves, which you can crush and apply to the infected area of your body. Once crushed, the leaves turn into pulp that serves as great treatment for boils when applied and the area bandaged.

Cabbage Treatment

Take a fresh leaf of cabbage and get rid of its ridges. Next, heat some water and then dip in the smooth leaf. Make the mixture into poultice form and apply it onto the affected area of the body.

It helps to wrap that part of the body with some loose bandage, with the poultice under it. Keep replacing the leaf material with fresh material until the abscess is diminished.

Echinacea Treatment

Extracts from the Echinacea herb can be applied to an area of the skin with abscess for the sake of eliminating inflammation and enhancing the function of the lymph system normally interfered with by bacterial infection.

The effectiveness of the Echinacea herb extract is thought to lie in the plant's potency in polysaccharides, which could be the active portions driving the external healing.

Besides fighting inflammation, Echinacea is also great at enhancing production of collagen and increasing hydration. These two effects are great at boosting the overall health of the skin and making it look bright.

Treatment of gingivitis & acne

Tea tree oil Treatment

Extracts from the tea tree can produce oil to be used in creams and gels, for the purpose of enhancing skin health. Essential oil from the tea tree can also be used when mixed with some carrier oil like the olive or coconut.

Jojoba Oil Treatment

Jojoba oil, which is waxy, is an extract from jojoba plant seeds. It helps to hasten healing of wounds, even those lesions that result from acne. The oil is generally great at repairing skin that has been damaged.

Among the reasons jojoba oil is great for skin health is that it has capacity to fight inflammation. As a consequence, it reduces the redness of the skin even as it reduces any pimple-related swellings. It also helps to eliminate whiteheads.

One of the ways you can effectively use the jojoba herb is to extract essential oil from it, and then incorporate it into a gel or cream, or even some clay mask for the face. All these products are great at eliminating acne.

Alternatively, you can put some jojoba oil drops onto some piece of cotton material, and then rub the oil-wet patch onto the part of the skin with acne.

Garlic Treatment

Garlic, which has been in use for centuries, is great at treating infections and boosting the body's capacity to decimate germs and fight infections.

The effectiveness of garlic lies in its richness in organo-sulfur compounds. These compounds not only have anti-bacterial but also anti-inflammatory properties. They are also great at boosting the body's immune capacity; hence keeping several ailments at bay.

Garlic is one of those herbal treatments easy to use, as you can simply incorporate it in your daily diet. If you choose, you can also chew the cloves, grind them and rub the matter onto bread, or even boil them in water and drink it as some hot beverage.

Note that applying garlic directly on skin is discouraged as it has potential to cause the skin some kind of burn.

Herbal Treatment for Allergies & Sinusitis

A person is said to experience some allergic reaction when his/her immune system gets triggered into overreacting to some allergen like pollen. If you are allergic to something, the moment you encounter it your body is bound to produce histamine, which is a chemical that initiates bothersome symptoms.

According to the CDC, or the US Center for Disease Control, it is possible to protect someone from reacting to an allergic trigger, although it is not easy to stop the allergy itself.

Although there are certain modern medications that inhibit histamine release, these often cause drowsiness and other unpleasant side effects. That is why many people are today seeking herbal treatments for allergies as opposed to buying over-the-counter anti-allergy medications.

Treatment of allergies

There are certain herbs that can prevent allergic reactions to people who have allergies. Extracts from these plants have capacity to prevent the body from releasing histamine; the substance responsible for causing allergic reaction.

Many of the anti-allergy herbs mitigate the symptoms of allergy, some of which appear on a seasonal basis. Use of herbs is preferred to the use of modern medicine as herbal medications are mostly free of side effects. Some of the prescription medicines given for the treatments of allergies often cause drowsiness; and some have more serious side effects.

Butterbur Treatment

The butterbur is an herb with reputation for effective treatment of migraines, but it also has capacity to treat certain symptoms of allergy. In fact, results of a scientific study carried in a British journal indicated that medication derived from the butterbur herb works just as effectively as cetrizine. However, the herbal medication does not cause the fatigue or drowsiness one is likely to experience after taking cetrizine.

Garlic Treatment

Garlic has also been found to contain quercetin; a substance credited with reducing the amount of histamine in the system.

Garlic is particularly important in the treatment of seasonal allergies because in spring the level of histamine in the body often rises, and the body goes on an overdrive in an attempt to fight the allergy-causing substances – allergens. The fact that quercetin is naturally present in garlic makes the herb well suited to fight allergies.

Other herbs great at preventing or treating allergies include stinging nettle, turmeric and rosemary.

With the stinging nettle herb, the leaves are the part relevant to allergy treatment. When cooked and consumed, the nettle leaves can actually offer protection against different forms of inflammation.

Treatment of sinusitis

People with sinusitis ordinarily have the problem marked by inflammation within their nasal passage, specifically on their mucus membranes. In addition, there is congestion of the sinuses that can sometimes be temporal.

When such congestion lasts only a few weeks, like below four weeks, the condition is referred to as acute sinusitis.

In case such becomes lasts for a period three months or longer, the condition is referred to as chronic sinusitis.

Sinusitis can be caused by viral or bacterial infection; and either kind has the impact of damaging the hair cells that line the sinuses.

Sometimes people develop sinusitis owing to exposure to allergens, which include pollen and dust, as well as coldness and smoke.

Another cause of sinusitis, though rare, is a defect of the sinus anatomy. Such a defect can adversely affect the septum in the nasal passage, cause enlargement of that passage, or develop nasal polyps.

One way you can suspect you are developing sinusitis is if you are persistently sneezing, especially the way a person does when with common flu. This condition is subsequently underlined by nasal congestion, which is accompanied with a running nose that produces yellowish-green phlegm.

When sinusitis is serious, you may develop fever and a cough; or even aches within the forehead and general facial area, or have your senses of smell and perception impaired.

The Ageratum Treatment

The ageratum herb is a flowering plant, which though ordinarily annual, sometimes becomes perennial. The flowers of the ageratum flower any time from the spring season up to fall.

The ageratum herb comes in numerous species, one of the most popular being the ageratum conyzoides.

This herb is used in the treatment of sinusitis when people drink it on a daily basis. You can wash the plant in its fresh form, measuring around 30 grams of it. It is recommended that you use water that is slightly salted for the washing, and then drain out the water before crushing the herb.

The alternative to fresh ageratum conyzoides is the dried form of the herb; and this is effective in a lesser amount – around 15 grams. If you mix this amount with 200 milliliters of water, and drink this mixture two times every day prior to taking meals, you will notice the symptoms of sinusitis diminishing.

Herbal Remedies for Bad Breath, Heartburn, GERD & Reflux

Sometimes people develop unpleasant breath, a condition referred to as halitosis, owing to the type of food they eat. This is especially so when there are particles of food around the area of the teeth. Such food remnants end up breeding bacteria, and those are responsible for the bad odor.

Other causes of unpleasant breath include smoking and use of other tobacco products; improper dental hygiene; consistent drying of the mouth; certain medications; and even mouth infections.

Nasal and even throat infections can also cause bad breath.

As for heartburn and the acid reflux, they can develop after consuming some types of foods or drinks. For example, coffee and alcohol; or bites like tomatoes, chocolate or other spicy foods can lead to heartburn or acid reflux. Even fatty foods can sometimes cause lead to such unpleasant health conditions.

Very often people develop heartburn and acid reflux when they have issues of obesity, or when they are under lots of stress. Other times this happens when the individuals are under certain medications like ibuprofen, which is a painkiller with capacity to fight inflammation.

Gastroesophageal Reflux Disease

The abbreviation for the Gastroesophageal reflux disease is GERD. It is a health condition that occurs when the muscle mass surrounding the base of the esophagus malfunctions.

Ordinarily during swallowing, this muscle band relaxes to facilitate the flow of food through and into the stomach. However, people with GERD have their stomach acid flowing back into the mouth, and this continues to persistently happen. For this acid to pass through, the esophagus will have permitted allowed it.

Permitting reversal passing of substances through the esophagus ends up causing heartburn and acid indigestion; and it is very easy for the individual to find it hard to swallow. Among the feelings such a person experiences is of food being stuck within the throat.

Among the causes of GERD are smoking and consuming massive meals before bed.

Best Herbs for Great Breath

There are certain natural remedies you can use to treat bad breath, many of which are herbal based.

The specific ailments that can cause unpleasant breath are chronic bronchitis, or diabetes when the person is not making an effort to control it. Others include use kidney conditions, disorders of the digestive system, RTIs or respiratory tract infections, or even GERD.

However, it is important to note that for many people, foul breath emanates from the mouth owing to inappropriate hygiene, dry mouth or even periodontal ailments.

Even then, there are people whose foul breath is a result of bacteria thriving in areas of the mouth where oxygen is limited; like beneath the tongue or within gum pockets. The bacterial produces sulfur compounds that are volatile as exemplified by hydrogen sulfide, and these compounds are responsible for the foul smell in the mouth.

Black & Green Tea

Both black and green teas have polyphenols, which are compounds known for stopping bacterial growth. Since one of the causes of foul breath is proliferation of bacteria, inhibiting multiplication of such bacteria is a good way of solving the problem.

Tea Tree Oil & Other Essential Oils

There are essential oils you can use in mouthwash to keep your mouth free of bad breath, and these include the tea tree and lemon essential oils.

Any time you use a mouthwash with these kinds of essential oils, the volume of the sulfur compounds is reduced, and consequently the risk of developing foul breath. Peppermint essential oil is another of the oils credited with effectively fighting bad breath.

It is important to note that any mouthwash with some alcohol content would end up drying out your mouth; a factor that contributes to generation of bad breath. In short, you ought to restrict your oral hygiene to alcohol-free mouthwashes.

Chewable Herbs

Another effective way of keeping your mouth fresh is chewing of safe herbs like rosemary and parsley, many of which are popularly put into culinary use. Other effective herbs include spearmint and tarragon. For these herbs to clear any foul breath and leave your mouth smelling fresh, you may need to chew them for a minimum of a minute.

Vegetables in Stew Form

Some of the herbs great at keeping foul breath at bay are best consumed in soup form. These include cucumber and other vegetables. Alternatively, you could ensure to eat plenty of juicy fruits or drink lots of water.

The idea generally is to keep your body, and particularly your mouth, hydrated. This helps to keep your body in good balance; meaning it is unlikely to have excess of the compounds that generate bad breath.

Best Herbs to Mitigate Heartburn, GERD & Reflux

Anyone with a problem of heartburn should avoid consuming foods that are fatty and those that are spicy. This means minimising consumption of fried foods like French fries.

Such people should also avoid coffee and drinks of the carbonated type, such as cola, and also alcohol. It is also advisable to avoid fruits like citrus, and vegetables like garlic or onions. It is also best to avoid consuming tomato sauce and chocolate.

Still, there are herbs that you can rely on to minimize incidences of GERD, and these include peppermint, ginger root, caraway, lemon balm and turmeric; garden angelica, licorice root and milk thistle; as well as the greater celandine and flowers of the German chamomile.

One important thing to keep in mind is that peppermint does not go together with anti-acids; and doing so could aggravate a heartburn situation.

As for the ginger root, not only is it great at reducing heartburn, but it is also effective in suppressing GERD. This is because with its great anti-inflammatory capacity, it is effective in reducing the swelling and even irritation that develop in the esophagus during GERD.

It is also important to note that the ginger root should also not be consumed in excess, as doing so could initiate or aggravate heartburn.

BOOK 10

NATIVE AMERICAN

HERBAL GARDEN

CHAPTER 1

HOW TO GROW HERBS IN LITTLE SPACE

Undeniably, it is expensive to do farming on vast land, but it is possible to grow herbs in a small space. People need to understand first that fresh herbs do not only provide natural harmless treatments; they also bring fragrance to your living area.

One convenient way of growing herbs when you are constrained in space is using pots. Many people have already learnt the method of growing herbs for culinary use in pots; plants such as basil and chives that are very popular with baked potatoes. You can use this same technique to grow herbs for medicinal use.

Factors to Consider

If you decide to grow herbs in one restricted area, you need to choose those herbs whose water requirements and need for sunshine are similar.

Of course it may be necessary to use different pots for different herbs because it may become necessary to supplement the soil for certain herbs with specific nutrients not important to other herbs.

Sometimes having separate pots for different herbs makes it convenient to move select pots around, either to be closer to or farther from direct sunshine.

In short, you can be self-reliant when it comes to medicinal herbs even when you live in an apartment or such other place where space is limited.

You can use your balcony or some little space outside your house to place pots like those used to grow flowers. Alternatively, you could place a polythene sack next to your window and plant the herb or herbs of your choice.

With this nature of knowledge, it is possible to grow even wild yams, tubers known to have a positive impact on the balancing of hormones known to mitigate conditions such as low libido and dryness of the vaginal area.

If the herbs you want to plant have massive roots that require relatively large space, these are best planted in individual pots rather than in polythene bags.

Principally, all your green plants need is sunlight, carbon dioxide and water, so that the process of generating their food, which is known as photosynthesis, can take place.

Integrity and Safety in Getting Medicinal Herbs & Seeds

As you grow your herbs, you need to ensure the area climate is conducive for these herbs to flourish.

If your plan is to use seeds for propagation, the popular technique is to put those seeds in some container that has water; and this is for purposes of germination.

When your herbs are ready for use and you decide to pick some for use, you can store them safely by immersing the plant stems as well as the leaves in jugs with fresh water. You need to avoid making use of pots, whether made of clay or glass, which are broken to grow your herbs.

As for watering of the herbs, this is appropriate only if the soil where the herbs are growing is dry. Otherwise, excessive moisture is normally not safe for herbs.

Washing & Drying of Herbs

Herbs need to be washed and well dried before storage. In fact, the ideal procedure is to wash and dry them as soon as you bring them into the house.

This is because the dirt and the bacteria on the surface of the herb can initiate the herbs' deterioration and accelerate it so that they are of little benefit to you.

It is normally recommended you wash your herbs under running water, and then lay them on some clean kitchen towel. This towel is meant to help you dry the herbs by patting them as they lie within the towel.

Another technique of preparing your herbs before storage is using some salad spinner to squeeze out a significant portion of the moisture.

Storage of Tender Herbs for Short Durations

If your herbs are the tender type and you intend to use them before long, you need to clip their bases off the stem even as you eliminate any leaves that have wilted or turned brown.

Once prepared in this manner, the next step recommended is to place them inside some mason jar or such like container. Even a glass jar ordinarily meant for water can be used to hold such herbs.

Just ensure you pour a little amount of water in the container, roughly one inch from the bottom of the container. The idea is actually to put the same amount of water normally put in a jar of fresh flowers.

If your jar or container has a lid, it is fine to cover the herb-holding container. You need to store the jar in the refrigerator until such a time as you are ready to use the herbs.

For any herbs stored in the refrigerator, it is crucial that you replace the water after every few days.

Storage of Tough Herbs for Short Durations

For herbs that are comparatively hardy, you can just store them in the refrigerator without having to immerse them in water. Instead, it is recommended that you wrap these in some paper towel, ensuring the towel is damp; and thereafter to wrap them in some plastic material.

Long-term Storage of Tender Plants

For herbs that are tender, such as basil, you may need to blend them alongside a few tablespoons of olive oil, or even canola oil, if you intend to keep them for long.

You can them put the blended herbal material in the normal trays for ice-cubes. The next step is then to put these trays in some freezer bag. This way, you can easily extract the portion of herb you need from the tray, leaving the rest intact and still frozen.

It is important to note that use of oil when blending your tender herbs is not mandatory. You can use water if you so wish.

Also, in case there are no ice-cube trays available for use you can chop the herbs and put them directly in your freezer bag. Soon after, add in either some oil or even water, and after mixing the matter embark on squeezing out the moisture. After you have squeezed out all the moisture you are able to lay the freezer bag flat and leave it.

Herbs prepared in this manner can last in their frozen form for many months with no risk of developing any greenish slime.

Long-term Storage of Hardy Plants

If you want to keep your hardy plants for a long period, you can freeze them the same way you store foods.

Wrap them well like a burrito and then secure them in some freezer bag; ensuring to label the bag for purposes of identification.

In fact, you can divide your herbs into smaller portions each of which you wrap separately with plastic wrappers, and then insert all of them together in some freezer bag. The benefit of dividing herbs in this manner is that you only unwrap the portion of herbs you need at any one time.

Mark you this method is cost-effective as the freezer bags you put your herbs in and seal are reusable.

CHAPTER 2

HOW TO TAKE CARE OF AN

HERBAL GARDEN

Just like other plants, the weather conditions need to be appropriate for medicinal herbs to thrive. It is important to know if the herbs of your choice are sensitive to either high temperatures or intense cold, so that the gardening effort you make can bear fruit. For some herbs, excessive cold could harm them, while for others extreme heat could scorch them dead.

How to Identify the Right Weather to Plant an Herb

According to gardening experts, temperatures that range from 65°- 70° Fahrenheit during the day are ideal for majority of herbs. In terms of Celsius, this range is 18° to 21°. For night-time, the ideal range of temperatures is said to be 55° – 60° Fahrenheit or 13° to 16° Celsius.

General Recommended Range of Temperatures

For basil, it is recommended that you grow it under temperatures that range from 65° to 85° Fahrenheit, or 18° to 29° Celsius.

For caraway, the recommended range of temperatures is 60° to 65° Fahrenheit, or 15° to 18° Celsius.

The temperatures ideal for the growth of chives range from 60° to 75° Fahrenheit, or 15° to 24° Celsius.

For cilantro, otherwise known as coriander, the best temperature range is from 60° to 70° Fahrenheit, or 15° to 21° Celsius.

The ideal range of temperatures for the herb, dill, is 70° to 85° Fahrenheit, or 21° to 29° Celsius. This is the same range of temperatures for lavender.

Meanwhile, the best range of temperatures for licorice and mint is 65° to 70° Fahrenheit or 18° to 21° Celsius, and 55° to 70° Fahrenheit or 13° to 21° Celsius respectively.

The ideal range of temperatures for the oregano herb is 55° to 70° Fahrenheit or 18° to 21° Celsius, and it is the same for rosemary.

The best range of temperatures for sage is 70° to 85° Fahrenheit, or 21° to 29° Celsius, while that of thyme is 60° to 75° Fahrenheit or 15° to 24° Celsius.

Meanwhile, the best range of temperatures under which to grow the yarrow is 70° to 85° Fahrenheit, or 21° to 29° Celsius.

How to Prepare Your Own Fertilizer & Manure

There are simple ways of making manure from where you are, and just like the natural herbs, home-made manure is safe both for the plants and the environment.

For example, you can make your own manure to use in the place your herbs are growing by mixing the dirt from the poultry house with grass clippings, and then adding animal urine. Just ensure the urine is not too much, otherwise it may burn the roots of your plants.

For safe use of urine in manure, make the ratio of urine to water one to twenty. In any case, such dilution significantly lessens the stench from the urine. The reason urine is a critical component of your garden manure is that it is rich in nitrogen.

As for the grass component, it contributes soluble nitrogen that is great for plant health. The components mentioned here so far are utilized in the preparation of liquid fertilizer.

You can also make manure by mixing the dirt from the poultry house with grass clippings, and only adding a little water or none at all.

Recommended Sources of Medicinal Seeds

Whether you intend to use seeds, seedlings or cuttings for planting, it is crucial that you get material in a manner that is ethical.

You need to understand that seeds are of different kinds; usually categorized according to how they are acquired.

Cross-Pollination

Among the seeds produced through cross-pollination is the heirloom.

The Heirloom

The heirloom comprises the seeds considered the origins of all medicinal species. It is possible to identify unique traits in them, the main reason they a quantity of them has been preserved over time.

To produce more of these heirlooms, cross pollination of plants is allowed season after season. The fascinating factor is that their original genes have remained stable; meaning the original benefits of the herbs are still applicable.

One organization known as Seed Saver Exchange has volunteered to preserve these valuable seeds, and you can source planting seeds from them.

The Hybrid

Another category of cross-pollinated seeds is the hybrid. To produce hybrid seeds, pollination takes place between two species of plants. This process is often pre-planned, with the people concerned wishing to produce a plant with specific characteristics. The environment is set but the pollination itself occurs in a natural manner.

Open-pollination

Seeds produced from open-pollination are those whose pollination is facilitated by birds or insects, or other natural factors such as wind.

There is one company in the US known as Fedco Seeds, and it is known for producing plant hybrid seeds for purposes of improving quality and reliability. You can even source organic seeds from this company that was founded in 1978 for purposes of supporting traditional farming.

Other Seed Production Methods

Other seeds are produced by way of selection and natural mutation, while others are produced through hybridization that does not require actual seeds. For such seeds, cuttings may be used.

There are those whose traits you would like to retain, and there are others whose traits you would like to modify. You can either source hybrids from original seeds modified in a laboratory set-up, or you can modify your own original plants through methods such as grafting.

Note that all the methods described above are ethical, as they do not cause harm to either people or the environment.

CHAPTER 3

HERBS FROM THE WOODLAND FIT FOR THE HOME SHADE

You may wish to understand why it is important to nurture woodland herbs, and perhaps you may be inspired to participate in their survival.

First of all, when you grow healing herbs in your environment, a close connection is created between your own systems and those of the plant fraternity. This connection becomes stronger as you continue seeing, smelling and even feeling the plants, as different seasons come and go.

Many of the woodland herbs used for medicinal purposes are also great for culinary use; and so you get to use them on almost on a daily basis.

It is important to try and cultivate woodland herbs especially those rare ones used as sources of medicine, because these could be at risk of extinction through acts of modern development.

Another reason it is important to cultivate medicinal woodland herbs is that not only do they offer much beneficial shade within the living environment, but they also divert people from going to harvest herbs from their natural habitats. In short, wildcrafting declines when people have cultivated their own herbs; the risk of over-harvesting is minimized.

It should be encouraging to know that cultivating woodland herbs is easy; even easier than growing normal food crops. If you have the right information, you will be able to prepare your woodland herbs in a manner that they may thrive on their own in a year or two. This means after one or two years; your woodland herbs may need very little input from you.

Embellishing Forests with Herbs

A forest where you introduce or add woodland herbs soon has great foliage and beautiful flowers that add to the richness of that forest. Herb pollination is enhanced and the soil is continually made richer.

Forests that can benefit from introduction of woodland herbs include those ordinarily preserved for their beauty, retention of water and to serve as animal habitats. When herbs are introduced or added and the existing forest biodiversity is enhanced, benefits accrue for both the people and the eco-system.

How to Grow Black Cohosh and Other Woodland Herbs

If your cultivation of woodland herbs is to succeed, you need to first know how to germinate the seeds. It is important also that you psyche yourself to be patient because patience is just as vital as the cultivation skills you exercise in nurturing these medicinal herbs.

Nevertheless, if time is a hindrance, you may choose to source ready-made seeds from firms that prepare them.

What Seed Stratification Entails

Seeds can naturally detect the changing of seasons; the cold or the hot; or winter transitioning to summer via autumn. When cultivating woodland herbs, you need to understand how to simulate these seasons so that the plants can respond in growth accordingly.

If you want the herbs to sense winter, you should have a way to create an environment of moisture and intense cold. One of the techniques you can use is creation of a controlled environment inside Ziploc bags, where you insert your seeds for germination. Germination seems to succeed better when stratification is done indoors.

Helpful Tips for Seed Stratification

The manner of seed stratification can also be cold-conditioning, where the seeds are exposed to extreme cold to simulate the cold winter conditions.

You need to assemble some amount of sand and then make it moist so that it is clearly wet; while ensuring no excessive water drips through even if the sand is squeezed.

In the absence of sand, you can also use organic material, as long as you ensure that material is not contaminated with fungal spores or any bacterial that can attack your seeds. The best material to use is one whose color is light; as opposed to using dark colored organic matter.

Put the planting material you choose in some small-sized Ziploc bag, after wetting the material, and then add in your seeds. The amount to put in your bag should measure around two or three tablespoons.

Mix the wet sand or organic matter and the seeds within the bag, and ensure those seeds are fairly distributed. The importance of such even distribution is that every seed will equally benefit from the moisture within the Ziploc bag.

Finally, label your Ziplog bag and put it inside one of the popular brown paper bags; the purpose of using the brown bag being to secure the seeds away from light.

Next, you need to store that brown bag in your refrigerator, and let it remain there for a minimum of three weeks and a maximum of three months. The duration should be dependent on the species of seed you are propagating.

In case you are not certain how long your seeds should remain in the refrigerator, try leaving them for a month before removing them.

When it is time to do the actual planting of the seeds, you can opt to pull out the seeds individually and plant them as such, or you can choose to plant them as they are with the body of sand or organic matter surrounding them. Of course, if the seeds are particularly large you would need to plant every seed separately.

Still, it is possible to stratify herbal seeds in a forest environment; meaning no transplanting will be required. Although this method of seed propagation may be relatively easier than planting indoors, it comes with challenges of seeds being eaten by animals like rodents before they can germinate, and rotting from the uncontrolled environment.

Others may also be infected by disease and die. Still, other seeds may succeed in germinating but their seedlings end up getting lost amidst other vegetation; in which case they cannot be nurtured for future use as medicinal woodland herbs.

One safe way of propagating woodland seeds outdoors would be using seed trays with reasonable depth. The tray can then be put on a cloth spread somewhere on the ground and the seeds left to germinate. Alternatively, the tray with seeds can be put inside a greenhouse with no artificial heating.

The herbs best propagated in this manner are mainly those that take long to germinate, like two or even three years. Good examples include the blue cohosh, scientifically known as *Caulophyllum thalictroides*, and goldenseal, whose botanical name is *Hydrastis Canadensis*.

Examples of herbal seeds that need to be stratified for them to germinate well include ginseng, black cohosh, bloodroot, goldenseal, trillium, wild yam and wild ginger, and the false unicorn root.

BOOK 11

HERBAL REMEDIES FOR CHILDREN

CHAPTER 1

HERBAL TREATMENTS FIT FOR KIDS

Children can also benefit from herbal treatments, which is a good thing because these treatments are unlikely to introduce complications or side effects to the child the way over-the-counter medications do.

We are speaking of the OTC medications because using herbal medications should not deter you from taking your child for his/her routine medical checkup, or to consult a specialist when your child is in agony.

Nevertheless, it is highly recommended that you have some herbal remedies for children within reach, because these will serve as your first aid kit whenever some unexpected medical incident occurs. And just like in cases of modern medicines, sometimes you do not need to take your kid to the hospital because the herbal treatment will have solved your child's problem.

Popular Herbs Safe for Kids

The commonest herbs considered safe for use by children include lavender, aloe vera, lemon balm, neem, thyme, marigold, garlic, peppermint, parsley, and rosemary.

Lavender Products

Although there are different ways lavender can be consumed, it is best to give it to children in form of tea. Lavender tea for kids helps them enjoy a good night's sleep.

Another great way to use lavender as kids' treatment is in form of oil. Lavender oil is helpful when used in a body massage.

If there is excess oil remaining the parents can use it to treat their hair, as it has properties that enhance hair health and growth. Adults can also use the oil for aromatherapy.

When you use lavender based herbal products on your children, they help to relieve these kids of any tension they may be feeling, even as they enhance the kids' clarity of mind.

These lavender based natural products also help to relieve headaches, even those as serious as migraines.

Besides pain relief, lavender is also great at mitigating respiratory issues in children. Also where physical grooming is concerned, you can rely on lavender based products to enhance the health of your children's skin and even their hair.

Aloe Vera Products

It is advisable that every parent or guardian have some aloe vera plants nearby because the plant is very handy with regard to emergencies such as wounds and sunburns. The soothing properties of aloe vera have the capacity to treat such health complications.

Although the aloe vera plant can thrive in varied weather conditions, it does best in areas with tropical conditions.

If your child has heartburn, a drop of the aloe vera sap can do him/her a lot of good. The reason aloe vera is great at clearing heartburn is that the toxicity level of this plant is very low.

Owing to its richness in Vitamin C, the aloe vera sap can be added to water to make a mouthwash fit to keep plaque at bay.

Also, any child consuming juice from the aloe vera plant remains safe from type 2 diabetes, as the plant has capacity to lower the level of glucose in the blood. The appropriate dosage is a tablespoon or two per child daily.

Parents and guardians can also make use of aloe vera in preserving children's fruits as well as vegetables. This plant has capacity to inhibit the growth and development of bacteria that would otherwise destroy the fruits or vegetables.

Lemon Balm Products

The lemon balm herb has capacity to reduce a child's anxiety, and even to lower a child's level of stress. Obviously, children who suffer from anxiety and whose stress levels are high cannot lead healthy lives.

Some of the best ways to serve lemon balm to children is to incorporate it into ice creams during preparation, or even in tea.

Once your child has consumed a product rich in lemon balm, his/her nervous system is soothed, and the children becomes relaxed with no disturbing fears or anxieties.

Another role lemon balm serves that is very beneficial to children is warding off insects. For that reason, you can decide to diffuse lemon balm inside your home, or even in surrounding areas for the purpose of keeping irritating insects away.

Other common uses of lemon balm with regard to treatment for children include reduction of swellings on the skin, and treatment of cold sores.

Neem Products

Neem is a tree from which medicinal material can be extracted. It is great for children because of its bacteria killing capacity.

The plant has seeds whose oil is therapeutic, and which are also used in the making of medicinal soap.

Different parts of the neem plant are medicinal; and they include the white, frail flowers. Children can consume these flowers after they have been cooked, or after they have been dried completely and sprinkled on meals as a garnish.

Neem comes in handy for children with worms, or if they have been bitten by insects and need healing. Neem products are also great for children who have acne, or those whose parents want to eliminate some dark patches on the skin.

Also, neem leaves mixed with honey forms a paste that is effective in the treatment of boils in kids. This mixture can also fight ringworms and eczema, and other different skin illnesses of a mild nature. It is also great at quelling itching on the skin.

In case a child has redness in the eyes or is experiencing irritation in the eyes, you can boil neem leaves in water and then use that water after it has cooled to wash the child's eyes. You can do the same for a child whose eyes look tired for no apparent reason.

Thyme Products

Although thyme is famous for its culinary use, you can make children's mouthwash with it. This mouthwash is medicinal and comes in handy in treating any fungal or bacterial infections a child may have developed.

Also, consumption of thyme by children improves their immunity. It also enhances the children's blood circulation.

Thyme is also effective in the treatment of colds as well as sore throat in kids. It is generally good for enhancing the respiratory function in children.

The reason thyme is so effective in all these children treatments is that it contains a compound known as thymol, which is the active ingredient responsible for the healing.

Marigold for Children

Although children are bound to love the marigold flowers if you cultivate the plant, marigold is handy when it comes to enhancing the health of your kid's skin.

The flowers have skin healing properties because of their richness in antioxidants and other health components, and the plant in general has anti-bacterial as well as antiseptic properties.

You can also rely on the marigold flowers to repel insects, which would otherwise disturb your child.

Marigold also has capacity to fight inflammation, hence enhancing the health of your child's skin. It can also fight infections of the ear, and at the same time reduce any pain the child might be experiencing.

Garlic for Children

Garlic is another herb popular for its culinary value, but which is also great at treating children's illnesses. Just consuming food with garlic enhances the child's capacity to fight infections and other illnesses.

Another health value that comes with children consuming garlic is the control of cholesterol. In fact, considering that more and more children are experiencing the risk of high cholesterol due to modern eating habits, it is advisable to encourage children to eat garlic whenever there is an opportunity. In fact if they can manage, eating raw garlic is even better for their health.

Besides garlic being great at enhancing heart health by reducing cholesterol and lowering blood pressure, it also helps to enhance the digestive function.

Peppermint for Children

Peppermint is not only great for children because it enhances the taste of their popular gum; it is also has soothing properties that can help to relieve muscle aches in kids. You can also give your child peppermint if you are convinced he/she has a stomach problem, because not only does peppermint relieve aches, but it also fights nausea and enhances digestion.

Having the peppermint herb around the house is also convenient as the herb has capacity to fight allergies. It also fights foul breath owing to its anti-bacterial properties.

Parsley for Children

Besides parsley's culinary value, it is also great at boosting the immune system. You can also rely on parsley to improve your child's digestive function even as it strengthens the child's bones.

Parsley's health benefits mainly emanate from the fact that it is rich in Vitamin K, and it has antioxidant properties. These, plus other health components in the herb makes parsley one of the best herbs you need to have in your home for your children's sake.

Even if parsley is an effective healing herb when consumed in food, you can also make some juice from it, or brew some tea for your child to drink.

Rosemary for Children

Rosemary is another herb popular for its culinary use, but which is also effective and safe as a treatment for children.

Among the reasons Rosemary is effective as an herbal treatment is its richness in vitamins and minerals. These two help to enhance the child's body functions and to improve the child's normal growth.

For example, the herb has capacity to enhance children's memory, and also to enhance the growth of their hair. In fact, you can make tea from the Rosemary herb and give it to your child for purposes of mitigating a declining hairline.

Other health benefits of Rosemary to kids include enhancement of blood circulation, fighting inflammation, fighting foul breath, and enhancement of the liver function.

Rosemary is also credited with enhancement of a child's brain function.

Children's Immune Boosters

There are also some herbs you can introduce to your children even if they are not ill, for the purpose of enhancing their immunity.

These include the elderberry and Echinacea, as well as goldenseal. Others include Oregano and the Black Seed, from where you can extract oil and feed to your child.

CHAPTER 2

CHILDREN AILMENTS HERBS CAN TREAT

There are several ailments that lead parents to visit the pharmacy, but which can be treated using herbs available in North America and elsewhere. Among those ailments is a sore throat.

Kids' Physical & Mental Issues Herbs can Safely Treat

Although pharmaceuticals are not short of children's medications, some concerns persist regarding the side effects some have; some in the short-term, and others in the long-run.

For example, some of the syrups prescribed to children for treatment of colds make the children so drowsy that they cannot function normally. So, if they are of school-going age, they do not benefit much for the days they are on medication.

For this reason, it would be helpful to learn the natural treatments parents can rely on to treat their children without exposing them to unnecessary side effects.

Sore Throat in Children

Among the herbs most effective in the treatment of sore throat in children is the slippery elm, whose botanical names are either Ulmus Fulva or even Ulmus Rubra.

The medicinal extract from this tree comes from the inner part of its bark. This extract, otherwise termed the mucilage, is gummy, and it is the one that forms a slimy gel when water is added to it and the two are mixed together.

The effectiveness of this gel lies in its capacity to line the throat and the digestive tract, in a manner to coat the child's mucous membrane and to soothe it. This way, any potential cough is suppressed.

Sometimes extract from the slippery elm is dried and ground into powder form, and then orange juice is added to it to make its flavor more acceptable to children.

Children's Stomach Discomfort

Just like adults, children sometimes suffer stomach discomfort, and luckily there are herbs that can alleviate the problem. One of these herbs is ginger, which is also used as a spice.

Owing to ginger's capacity to stimulate generation of saliva, gastric secretions and bile in particular, it ends up mitigating problems that would otherwise lead to upset of the child's tummy.

Also, ginger has capacity to suppress contractions of the gastric area, and to improve the tone of the intestinal muscles as well as the peristalsis, which is the movement of the intestinal tract.

Taking ginger is advantageous to children as it is safe for them. They can even chew it raw if they experience nausea, and not only will the nausea disappear, but the child will be prevented from vomiting.

Just as in the use of garlic by children, fruit juice can be used to make the herb taste a little better. With the ginger root, you can boil it first and then add some apple juice to it before serving the drink to the child.

Another herb that is not only effective but also safe for children is chamomile. You can make tea from this herb and serve your child if he/she has some stomach discomfort. Chamomile is even more advantageous compared to other herbs because it is safe even for infants.

You can actually feed it to a baby with colic and its tummy troubles will end. It is important to note that chamomile is not only anti-inflammatory; it also has sedating properties. For that reason, it has capacity to reduce the movements within the child's small intestines. By so doing, any ache or even cramping the child might be experiencing is mitigated.

Another herb that is great at treating stomach upsets in children is peppermint. It even reduces stomachaches and pains in the abdomen.

Diarrhea & Constipation

Diarrhea is another ailment that plagues children. The same case applies to cases of constipation. Herbs, especially those with probiotics, are very important in replenishing the bacterial considered good for the body; which will have been flushed out through diarrhea.

The suitable herbs not only slow down the diarrhea, hence protecting the child from dehydration; but they also create and enhance health within the child's intestines.

Peppermint is one of those herbs you can use to enhance the health of your child's gut. It has capacity to reduce diarrhea and to reduce the symptoms associated with IBS, the health condition known as Irritable Bowel Syndrome. This herb also helps to solve the problem of constipation and cramping.

Besides incorporating peppermint into children's food or drinks, you need to feed them with foods rich in fiber; foods like raisins and prunes, or even dried fruit.

Earaches in Children

You can use herbs like the mullein plant to treat children's earaches. In the practice of modern medicine, doctors would use antibiotics when the aches are deemed to be the result of a bacterial infection.

However, you can put drops of oil from the mullein plant into your child's ear, and any inflammation will begin reducing. In due course, both the inflammation and accompanying irritation will disappear.

This is something University of Massachusetts's Chris Kilham, an expert in alternative medicine, concurs with.

The parts of the mullein plant with healing properties include the leaves, flowers and the roots; all of them having capacity to treat infections.

Other experts have found the leaves of the mullein plant to be effective in the treatment of tumors, and in fighting viral, bacterial and fungal infections.

Child Fever

One herb you can rely on to reduce your child's fever, if it has not reached dangerous levels, is tea made out of the ginger root while fresh. Such tea is rich in anti-microbial properties, and so if the fever is particularly accompanied by a cold or a condition like bronchitis, you can be certain the ginger tea will destroy the rhinovirus normally associated with colds.

Child's Mild Burn

In case your child gets a mild burn at home, you can use the aloe vera herb to soothe and cool it.

Nevertheless, there is an even better herb when it comes to treating burns, and that is the tamanu. The botanical name for this herb is Callophylum inophyllum, and the plant's oil has been recognized internationally for its capacity to create scar tissue for the sake of enhancing the burn's healing process.

Witch hazel is another plant that you can rely on for treatment of mild burns at home. The witch hazel is a tree from which ointments are made for the purpose of treating burns, particularly during emergencies. When you apply a witch hazel product on an area that has a mild burn, damage to the tissues is mitigated.

Bruises on Kids

If you find an inflammation or a bruising on your child, one of the best products you can apply to reduce damage to the body is a cream or a gel from the arnica plant. The arnica flowers comprise the plant part, which is potent with healing properties, which include the capacity to reduce swellings. Another name for the arnica herb is Montana.

ADHD

For parents whose children have been recommended Adderall or even Ritalin, both of which are strong pharmaceutical drugs, you may opt to try out the Rhodiola rosea herb instead. Rhodiola rosea is popularly known as the goldenroot or even the rose root.

The greatest advantage in the use of herbal treatments like Rhodiola rosea is that it does not introduce any risk of side effects, the way pharmaceuticals do. Today you may be able to find it packed in capsule or liquid form, or even sold as tablets for use by young kids.

Goldenroot has undergone numerous tests as researchers continue to find best herbs to substitute or complement modern medicines, and one factor that makes the herb stand out is its effectiveness on mental health while having no adverse side effects.

Children Allergies

Children are sometimes allergic to different things in the environment; things like pollen or grass. One of the best treatments for allergies is natural honey, and as it is obvious, a lot of the goodness of honey comes from the nectar they collect from plants.

However, parents and guardians should avoid feeding honey to infants, or babies less than a year old. Doing so might lead to the baby developing botulism, a gastro-intestinal health issue which, though rare, is actually serious.

What would happen in cases of infant botulism is bacteria emanating from spores ending up growing and multiplying within the infant's intestines; and this eventuality has the potential to produce hazardous toxins in the body.

Besides honey in its natural state, another natural remedy for children's allergies is saline. To make saline, all you need to do is mix a tablespoon of salt with a quart of cool boiled water. You can then squeeze a squirt or two in the child's nostrils.

This is great for reducing inflammation and also any irritation the child may have developed as an allergic reaction.

Hives & Rashes

Just like some forms of irritation and inflammation, rashes, and also hives, often develop as allergic reactions to external factors. Still, they can develop when a child becomes very nervous. A good example is when a child is about to go to a new school for the first time; whether a kindergarten or a new elementary school. Such a child might have hives breaking out.

Although no fresh herbs have not been directly recommended, there are natural products you can use on the child to mitigate the problem. For example, you can dissolve a cup of Epsom salt in warm water in a child's bathtub.

The reason hot water is inappropriate is that it may end up triggering additional histamines and hence exacerbating the hives or rashes. Also, the reason cold water is inappropriate for this purpose is that it has potential to close the pores on the child's skin, which in turn would reduce the child's capacity to absorb the much needed salt.

This information goes to show there are several ailments that can befall your child without any warning sign, but you need not rush to the pharmacy for solutions. In short, you can build an emergency kit of natural remedies right at home by ensuring you have herbs growing in your home environment.

BOOK 12
HERBALISM AND ALCHEMY

CHAPTER 1

CONTROL & REGULATION OF HERBAL REMEDIES

Regulation of herbal treatments may not be as standardized and stringent as that of modern medicine, but still there is a degree of regulation. Regulation is mostly meant to keep users of these medications safe from overdose and misplaced use. It is also meant to ensure there is continued vigilance so that information pertaining to contraindications with modern medicine is disseminated to the public as soon as it is available.

Among the organizations that play important roles in monitoring and exercising some form of regulation of pharmaceuticals across the world are the FDA or Federal Drug Administration; WHO or the World Health Organization, the EU or the European Union, and other organizations whose regulation is localized.

These same organizations have begun to take interest in the use of herbal products, not only because there may be replication of use when a person on prescription medicine takes herbal infusions, tea or such other product, but because people might act without adequate information.

For example, people with serious illnesses might mistakenly abandon their prescriptions and embark on treatments whose efficacy has not been proven.

The Role of WHO in Regulation of Herbal Treatments

WHO began practical ways of understanding the world of herbal medicine in 1992, the year the organization got some experts to develop appropriate principles by which research on and assessment of herbal treatments would be carried out.

The experts noted that herbal medications had an important role to play in the enhancement of people's health, and they acknowledged the need to monitor the efficacy and use of these treatments.

Besides acknowledging the role of herbal treatments in enhancing people's health, WHO also recognizes the importance herbal medicines have in the advancement of modern medicine. For that reason, the organization has continued to support the testing of these medications scientifically.

Nevertheless, there are several herbal treatments in use that have not yet undergone any scientific study, and people have generally relied on the positive outcomes observed over the years.

WHO ended up compiling guidelines on the use of herbal treatments in 1996; and these covered the quality and efficacy of the medications, as well as the safety of the users. According to WHO, the guidelines would help the organizations in charge of regulating medicinal drugs and their use to monitor producers of herbal medications, and to help them in documenting the components and other factors of their products.

One crucial point that was included in the 1996 guidelines pertains to the authority given to regulatory bodies to cancel licenses of pharmaceutical companies whose medicines included herbal ingredients with toxic effects.

The Role of the EU in Regulation of Herbal Treatments

As per the EU herbal treatment stipulations, every member state must seek approval before it can proceed to market any of its herbal products. EU has even provided a standard definition to its members, regarding what herbal medications mean. The EU spells out the compositions that are considered safe, acceptable plants, and product efficacy levels manufacturers are expected to observe.

Quality Control of Herbal Remedies

Every member of the EU is able to access a list of those herbal products acceptable for marketing within the EU; and these are products whose efficacy has been proven. Every one of those countries is expected to have a national body, which should ensure herbal products produced in the country are not only of high quality but also safe for use.

Such a body is expected to establish that some reasonable experimental regimen has been followed, in a bid to confirm the product's efficacy.

Processed Herbal Products

It is necessary for marketers of herbal products to have their products properly licensed before releasing them to the market, particularly if those products have been processed. If your firm is involved in the processing of such natural products, you need to ensure you have proof they have undergone clinical trials.

Imported Herbal Medications

Different EU countries have different forms of quality assurance when it comes to assessing the efficacy and safety of herbal products. In fact, different countries have leeway to follow different techniques in preparing their plant products.

However, for those herbal products that enter the market as raw materials, they are not subjected to regulatory measures like the processed and packaged products. Good examples are those plant products that enter the EU market in form of foodstuff. Nevertheless, any plant material that has been modified in one way or another needs to be checked for quality and efficacy, and very importantly, for safety.

BOOK 13

THE HERB MASTER'S TERMINOLOGY

CHAPTER 1

HOW TO BECOME A MASTER HERBALIST

You may be someone who has acquired knowledge of herbal remedies through observation and practice, or you may have been bequeathed the knowledge by your parents. However you found yourself practicing herbal medicine, you can still advance and become a master herbalist.

Becoming a master herbalist involves undertaking studies and taking advantage of herbal properties, all of which are natural, for enhancement of clients' health and overall wellbeing.

As a master herbalist, you are able to evaluate the lifestyle of your client, and to determine the individual's health needs.

Job Opportunities for Master Herbalists

You may need to understand that there are several opportunities to enhance people's health after achieving the status of master herbalist. Practicing as an individual herbalist is not the only opportunity.

You can work as a chiropractor, physiotherapist, or even as a food or herbal supplement expert.

Many master herbalists grow their own herbs, dry them, and even formulate their own herb-based products.

Beneficial as herbal products are, and informed as herbalists may be, the sector still have challenges. One of the biggest challenges master herbalists face is acceptance. It may take you a few years for your potential clients to believe you are credible enough to nurture their health.

The reason ordinary folk often have doubts regarding the competence of herbalists is lack of standardization of the practice by the state. Nevertheless, those who are patient enough to win people's confidence end up building a large population of loyal clients.

The easiest way to mitigate the challenge of trust today is to earn the credentials of a master herbalist. That way, people will feel reassured as they entrust their healthcare to you or your clinic.

Course Requirements

You need to pursue a degree course before you can quality as a master herbalist; meaning you should have first completed your secondary school course. Nevertheless, there are some universities that can admit you for the degree course on the basis of certain postgraduate certificates.

In some rare cases, some herbalists have been practicing for so long and have built so much credibility across communities that they are given opportunities to formalize their knowledge through university study.

The fields of study you need to pursue in order to attain a relevant degree are either herbal studies or clinical herbalism.

You also need to have had some experience of a clinical nature, which has been set as a basis for you to be admitted to the American Herbalists Guild or AHG.

Though voluntary, many master herbalists find it beneficial to acquire certification from the AHG.

Basic Units of Study

As far as academics and training are concerned, you need to be prepared to study human anatomy and biology; identification of plants; the history of herbal practice; the theory of herbalism; health enhancement through herbalism; herbalism and illnesses; and ethics of medical practice.

In fact, there are some topics that one cannot miss in the curriculum if pursuing a degree in herbal medicine. In addition to those whose units have been mentioned, others include endocrinology, chemistry, mathematics, herb history, herbalists of historical significance, world outlook to herbology and historical use of herbs by different cultures.

One must also study a minimum of a hundred medicinal herbs, and learn how to prepare tea and tinctures, and extract medicinal matter from them.

You can also expect to be taught how to identify individual herbs when they are still in the natural habitat; make use of herbs to detoxify the body; and use the herbs to strengthen body organs, both internal and external.

You are also taught how to differentiate between herbs of high quality from those not worth using; and where to source herb supplies if you are not cultivating your own.

Suffice it to say, by the time you complete your studies on herbal medicine, you will not only have gained invaluable relevant information, but also gained the confidence to begin practising as a master herbalist.

American Herbalist Guild Requirements

The credential you acquire after entering the register of qualified herbalists maintained by the AHG is RH, which stands for Registered Herbalist.

To acquire this credential, your learning and training in herbal medicine must have covered 4 years; and you also must show proof of practical experience of not less than 400hrs.

The number of patients you will have attended during this period should be 100 or more.

In addition to proof of training, length of hands-on practice and number of patients attended to, you need to prove you know and understand 150 herbal plants used for medicinal purposes, at the minimum.

All these requirements are in addition to those already mentioned like having understanding human anatomy, knowledge of plant chemistry, and being ethical as far as your professional practice is concerned.

You also need to present to AHG letters from three credible referees, recommending you for registration. On top of these recommendations, you need to present your own some case histories, the minimum number being three.

Gladly, the organization offers its certification online; meaning you can apply for registration from wherever you are.

Master herbalists may also be pleased to learn that AHG is not the only credible organization offering registration. There are others as well; and different herbalists may choose to register under certain bodies to match their own needs or those of their target clients.

Major Skills of a Master Herbalist

A qualified master herbalist is expected to be skilled not only in identifying herbs, but also in communication and analytical skills. The individuals also need to have a good understanding of the human anatomy and also physiology, and to have acceptable bedside manners.

Remuneration for Employed Master Herbalists

If you want to secure a job as a master herbalist, you may wish to know the state of the employment market. There is room to be absorbed in the US economy as a degree holder in the field of herbalism, and the remuneration as per 2019 statistics was slightly more than $75,000 per year.

Importance of Seeing a Client in Person

Often herbalists start their career by treating people familiar to them, and over time they build a sizeable number of clientele.

Although in this age of technology it is tempting to attend many clients over the phone, it is advisable that you endeavor to see your clients in person.

This is easy to understand if you consider a client who informs you he/she has a child whose stomach appears swollen and has been so for several months. If the consultancy is going on over the phone, you are likely to think of possible inflammations of the stomach; and that is the trajectory that will dictate the herbs to recommend.

However, if the client had brought the child along for you as the herbalist to assess him/her, you might probably notice that in addition to the child's stomach being distended, his/her hair has turned blonde and brittle.

With this personal observation, you may not give much consideration for herbs with antibacterial properties; but instead might consider herbs that would serve as dietary supplements for the child. This is because the symptoms you will have observed are associated with kwashiorkor, a health condition that comes about from poor eating habits.

In short, it is important to see your client as you listen to his/her health issues, because you are likely to pick up subtle details that would help you be more accurate with your diagnosis. On the contrary, the person explaining the patient's health condition to you might leave out some important details, mistakenly thinking they are of no consequence.

NOTE

As a qualified and confident herbalist, you should be free to cooperate with other experts in the health sector. This means if you treat a client and realize your skills or resources are limited in the context of the ailment you are facing, you should not hesitate to refer the client to a physician in a modern clinic.

There are even instances your intuition might dictate you refer the client to a hospital; like if the person presents with abnormally intense pain in some internal part of the body. You may also wish to do the same if a client informs you his/her extremely high fever has just set in without other accompanying symptoms.

In short, a good master herbalist should not feel incompetent if he thinks traditional treatment may not be adequate for his/her patient; and therefore finds it appropriate to refer the patient to a modern clinic or to a clinical doctor.

In fact, you are taught to maintain this mindset during training – that if, in your opinion, your patient requires further observation, tests or treatment, you should not hesitate to make the necessary referrals.

Whether your specialty is herbal or modern medicine, the fields should always be complementary and not competing.

How to Test for Herb Edibility

It is crucial that you ensure any herb you harvest for consumption, either as a food or medication is edible.

First of all as a general rule, leave alone any plant growing alone; it may not be easy to determine its edibility, or if it is the herb you are actually thinking about.

Still, for someone who has specialized in herbal medicine, it is not necessarily that difficult to identify edible herbs. The dandelions, the prickly pears, and such other edible plants are easy to identify.

Likewise, it is not necessarily difficult to tell if a plant is poisonous when you are moving through a natural habitat. Some signs that a plant has a high chance of being poisonous include being thorny, the plant grains having black spurs or purple ones sometimes, or the plant has spines.

Another way you can determine if the plant is poisonous is to sniff it, and if it smells like a poisonous plant you know then you can give it a wide berth. Generally, if the plant you sniff smells like almonds, then consider it to be toxic and leave it alone.

Universally Accepted Edibility Assessment

There are some techniques globally accepted for testing if a given herb is safe to consume. If your test gives you negative results, or even leaves you in doubt, you need to abandon the herb if still growing, or discard it if already harvested, so that you do not put anyone's health at risk.

Test by way of contact

Using this test involves you taking some piece of herb and rubbing it on a part of your body. The best areas on which to test an herb for edibility include the wrist on the inside area of your elbow.

Take a couple of hours before you can wipe off the herb residues or moisture from your skin, to give the substance time to react, if it should. Experts recommend 8hrs of waiting.

Logically, if you get a reaction on your skin after you have rubbed the plant on it, the same reaction can be expected inside your body if you ingest the herb. This is a sign the herb is not fit for consumption.

Dissect the Herb

The reason for dissecting the herb is to find out if the entire plant is healthy. It would be unfortunate to assume a plant is healthy and proceed to grind it, only to realize it had mould inside. So, split the herb into different parts, and check if it harbours any mold or worms, or even other parasites. An herb with rot or parasites should outright be discarded.

Test by Tasting

When using this technique, the piece of herb you bite should be very tiny and you should not hasten to swallow it.

You need to place a small piece in your mouth and wait a little while. If you sense some burning or even some tingling, you should categorize the herb as unfit for consumption; hence spit out the bit you had in the mouth. For your own safety, rinse off the taste immediately with clean water.

It needs to be mentioned that just because an herb does not taste nice to the palate does not mean it is poisonous. Many plants do not taste nice when raw.

The Cooking Test

With this technique, you need to bite the herb after boiling it. If you detect some stinging on your tongue or any part of the mouth, then you need to spit out the bit of herb and wash your mouth. Such stinging is normally a sign the plant is toxic. Obviously, unless you are at home, a campsite or such other location where fire is available, you may just contend with testing the herbs raw.

The Chewing Technique

Sometimes you may consider it necessarily to chew on the herb, if you do not experience any reaction when you put a piece in the mouth. The reason for chewing on the herb would be to find out if by chewing the herb it will release toxins. If it does, you will certainly sense some burning or tingling; hence classify the plant as unfit for consumption.

BOOK 14

HERBAL TERMINOLOGY FOR BEGINNERS

CHAPTER 1

EFFECTIVE AND SAFE USE OF HERBS

Native Americans realized ages ago how potent medicinal herbs were, and so they have been handling them as plants of great value; and also plants with potential to harm if misused.

Whereas they derived value from the plants through chewing, smelling or smoking, there are those like tobacco that they used not only for their own physical healing, but also as offering to their gods as a way of worshipping them. For instance, they would offer tobacco to the earth, which they considered their revered mother.

In the ancient days, herbs had not been commercialized, and if they had it is doubtful they would have managed to buy them considering they were not an affluent community.

Nevertheless, they knew how to pick valuable herbs where they grew wild. They would then use them in different ways; some for physical healing, others for cleansing environments deemed to be contaminated by bad spirits, or even to purify things meant for consumption or other use.

Plenty of the knowledge Native Americans had pertaining to natural herbs forms the basis of today's herbal practice. Within that knowledge are basic principles of herbal use.

Principles of Herbal Use

Note the Herbs to Avoid during Pregnancy

Avoid consuming herbs while pregnant unless you have assurance from your doctor these herbs are safe for the baby in the womb.

Risk of Premature Contractions

Some herbs like parsley or the willow may have some adverse effects on your pregnancy. In the meantime, herbs you need to avoid because of the risk of inducing premature contractions include the yarrow, and the cohosh family – black cohosh and negro. Others include the maidenhair fern, lady's mantle, angelica, shephard's purse, sacred bark, gotu kola, ergot, male fern, devil's claw, hops, golden seal, St. John's Wort, juniper berry, motherwort, bugleweed, zoapatle, passion flower, yohimbe, buckthorn, rhubarb, rue, feverfew, clover, fenugreek, pastora and cat's claw.

Other Risks

There are other herbs you need to avoid when pregnant because of diverse reasons, like toxicity, neuro-toxicity or being hallucinogenic; being abortifacient or toxic to the liver; being outright poisonous; or being unfit for ingestion.

These include the aloe vera, wormwood, cassia, cinnamon, moonflower, wormseed, Mexican tea, fennel, pennyroyal, tobacco, basil, oregano, Boldo, castor oil, rosemary, comfrey and corn smut.

Only use Herbs whose Properties you Know

Just because you have learnt that herbs are of medicinal value does not mean it is alright to use herbs haphazardly.

Nevertheless, if you have not formally studied herbal medicine but have an understanding how the Native Americans used a particular herb, you can apply that information for your health benefit.

Danger lies in using herbs whose characteristics and potency you have no idea, because you risk using herbs that can become disastrous to your health or outright fatal.

Avoid using excessive number of herbs concurrently. If your intention is to rely on herbal treatment, the principle you should follow is one of one herb at a time. Once you apply the one you have chosen, or ingested it, you need to wait a while to take note of how your body is responding.

Spacing herbs when using more than one helps you understand the herb that is most helpful to you under the circumstances. It also helps you avoid mixing herbs in a manner that can be detrimental to your body.

If Native Americans shunned it, leave it too

You need to avoid using any herb that Native Americans did not use. There must be good reason why they avoided it.

In this regard, you even ought to stick with the particular use Native Americans used every herb for. This means if they used a given herb to treat inflammation by applying its extract on the skin, you should not try to ingest it instead; just stick to external use.

Avoid Ingesting Unless You Are Certain It Is Safe

Even though there is a wide range of herbs considered medicinal and safe for use, their safety extends only to its correct usage. So, if you are not certain a particular herb is edible, do not consume it.

For example, arnica flowers are great for topical use, meaning you can rub them on your skin and experience relief when sore or bruised; but eating them, unless in very tiny quantities, can lead to extremely bad poisoning.

Consume Herbs in Moderation

Good as herbs are, they need to be consumed in moderation. There are some that cause nausea and even vomiting when consumed in plenty.

If you are using a given herb for treatment, you may wish to begin with a little amount first, and probably increase as you deem necessary. Sooner or later you are going to establish the right amount and keep to it whenever you have the same health issue.

You need to do similar experiments for the sake of establishing how regularly you can consume the herb without feeling bad from its effects. In short, you need to establish the most suitable amounts are regularity; and that way you minimize the risk of nausea or vomiting.

Only use Herbs when in Balance

This means you should avoid consuming herbs if you feel your mind is not in the right place.

For you to be in the right state of mind, you need to be feeding well, meaning eating a balanced diet; and engaging in regular exercise, albeit mild. The right food combined with exercises keeps your body in good balance; a state necessary for healing. In short, herbs work best in the right body and mental environment.

Keep to Your Dosage

Once you have established the amount of herb that effectively and safely treats a certain ailment, use that amount every time you are ill. This includes maintaining the regularity you have established to be appropriate.

If the amounts of herb you consume are haphazard, you could find yourself taking too little sometimes, or spacing your doses too far apart, and concluding the herb is not effective for you.

Conversely, if the times of day you take the herbs are too close, or the amounts of herb you are consuming are massive, you may develop nausea, pains or other unfavorable responses, because essentially you will have overdosed.

How to Avoid Abusing Herbal Remedies

It is indisputable that today many people are self-medicating with herbs. While a good number of these people have acquired reasonable knowledge regarding the herbs' benefits following generational usage of traditional medicines, some simply follow the hype.

Unfortunately, without knowing if an herb has potential to cause harm and to what extent, herb users may end up putting their health in jeopardy. For that reason, it is important for you to read informative material pertaining to edible herbs and their safe use, and also how to avoid dangerous herbs. Books like this one are invaluable if people are going to benefit from use of herbs without putting their lives in danger.

Also, since there is a lot of information available all around regarding herbs as an alternative to modern medicine, it may be confusing to a layman and sometimes misleading. That is why you need to know the crucial facts within the realm of herbalism before deciding if a particular herb is good for use.

Check for Interactions

One such fact is that medicinal herbs can also be fatal; but that is if they are not used appropriately. According to hepatologist, Tatyana Kushner, a specialist doctor in liver conditions at Icahn School of Medicine, poor use of herbs can cause the liver function to fail, even to the extent of the person requiring liver transplant.

Mind the Dosage

Other experts have also warned on dangers of using too much herbal supplements, or even using them when you should not.

For example, while the St. John's Wort herb may be effective in the treatment of anxiety and sleep disorders, it bears the danger of interacting with several medications. The *Journal of Alternative and Complementary Medicine* in 2014 indicated that some levels of St. John's Wort used alongside some anti-depressants or drugs with blood thinning properties can put the person's life in danger. It may also reduce the effectiveness of birth control medications.

Follow the Correct Usage Technique

It matters a lot how you use a given herb. If you ingest an herb that is meant solely for external use, you could injure some vital organs. For that reason, it is important to understand how the particular herb was initially used by the original users; like the Native Americans. Through practice, they had learnt the safest way to make use of specific medicinal herbs.

In fact, people who have become herbalists by way of inheriting the tradition are encouraged to pass on the knowledge to their heirs; and where possible to document the information. They should also do the same about any ancient culinary and medicinal recipes they have.

Refer Serious Injuries to Hospital

Great as herbal medications are, there are some injuries or level of illnesses beyond their capacity to treat. For instance, a broken rib needs to be handled in a medical theater, a facility normally not available in herbalists' clinics.

Another good example of cases requiring referrals are ailments you have tried to treat for several months without reasonable improvement. In short, you need to keep remembering that your herbal practice and modern hospitals offer complementary services; all for the sake of enhancing people's health.

For that reason, whatever one party can do to make the other succeed should be done.

BOOK 15

THE LOST BOOK OF
ASTRAL HERBS

CHAPTER 1

NATIVE AMERICAN ASTRAL HERBS & THEIR USE

For you to understand how herbs can help in astral projection, you need to understand first what astral projection is.

Astral projection is best described as some out-of-body experience, which is often abbreviated as OBE. Individuals experience this state in their own unique way; and this should not be surprising considering this experience involves a person being in touch with his/her own spiritual existence.

On a day-to-day basis, the experience you normally have is that of your own body and how it is functioning. You are often interested in whether the body is well nourished in terms of the basic food nutrients like protein, minerals and the rest. However, when things go astral, it means you are no longer visualizing yourself in the physical state, but in the realm of the spirits.

Traditionally, it is believed every person has a spiritual existence as well; one that needs to remain healthy if the individual's health is going to be wholesome. This belief is still widely held.

When you are in this process of astral projection, you may be able to interact with other beings in the spiritual form, and get to understand issues you hardly understand when in your bodily state.

One crucial point to note is that although the astral world is that of spirits, you do not practically lose your bodily form. What you do is have capacity to project beyond your physical environment; hence embarking on a journey that traverses the mental realm and reaches a higher form.

Although to the uninitiated astral projection might come across as a dream, it is not. In fact, you can experience astral projection even when you are not asleep. It is even possible to induce this process after reasonable practice, so that you are able to transition into that higher realm when you wish. Ordinarily this requires dedicated and passionate focussing, beyond that which is required in normal meditation.

What has so far been explained is the traditional way of undertaking astral projection. In this chapter, you are going to learn how certain herbs can help you experience astral projection.

Herbs that Help Induce Astral Projection

In explaining their experience, many who have experienced astral projection note there is a silvery cord that links their physical body to the astral sphere; and this makes you feel safe during the experience. The connection you view reassures you that you are not held hostage; that you will be able to return to your normal world when you wish. This tells you astral projection is far from being a scary experience.

Traditionally, Greeks and Egyptians were known to engage in astral projection because they were curious to find out how the world beyond the physical looked and felt like.

It is important to note that the religious practice known as shamanism is based on astral projection. In shamanism, the practitioner has capacity to communicate with the spiritual world.

In fact, it is in this religious practice that the practitioner manages to direct helpful spiritual energy from its place of dwelling to the physical realm, for the purpose of having someone healed.

Energies of this nature also help practitioners in their quest to forecast matters, a feat one can only attain through divine intervention.

One needs to understand that when a shaman is actively at work, he/she assumes a state totally different from that people know; his/her consciousness rising to a higher level. To the eyes of those around, the shaman will have entered into a trance.

Shamans have professed gaining capacity to communicate with powers higher than normal, from which they receive guidance on challenging matters. These powers also give the shamans clarity in their endeavors, which in turn makes their work more effective. When it comes to treating people, shamans attribute their healing prowess to the higher powers.

Wormwood or Artemisia absinthium

If you find the wormwood in North America, take it to be one of those herbs with foreign origin. They originally grew in Asia and Europe, as well as North Africa. Today you can find this herb from the daisy family even in temperate regions of the globe.

The wormwood is not only herbaceous but also perennial, and you can identify it with its smell of sage that is particularly strong.

It is not surprising that this herb possesses astral capabilities, considering traditionally the Europeans used it to help them with their capacity to remember and perceive things; and even to think.

Even as it enhances people's mental capacity, the wormwood herb can also give them powerful psychoactive effects.

It is good to note that the effect of the wormwood has been acknowledged even in the commercial world, and manufacturers of pillows have begun to use its ingredients. In recommending these pillows, their manufacturers cite the capacity the herbal ingredients have, to enhance the lucidity of a dreamer and to make his/her dreams more vivid. Essentially too, the ingredients from the wormwood make it easier for the pillow user to undertake astral projection.

Huckleberry or Ericaceae

The huckleberry is actually a shrub native to America. Traditionally, it has thrived in both continents; North and also South America. In fact, natives of British Columbia were among the first communities to appreciate this herb for its edibility and medicinal value.

This herb that you can identify from its tiny and round berries, nevertheless, resemble big blueberries. The diameter of the berries ranges from five to ten millimeters.

The healing properties of the huckleberry herb include enhancing the relaxation and clarity of the mind; a development very paramount when it comes to astral projection.

The Bakana Herb

The Bakana plant, whose origin is Mexico, contributes greatly in enhancing the experiences associated with astral projection; visualizing yourself out of body.

Besides enhancing your out-of-body experience, the Bakana can also relieve you of pain. This herb has also been associated with treatment of some forms of mental illness.

The Valerian Root or Valeriana officinalis

The Valerian herb is a perennial herb that originated in Rome and even Greece. Its enhancement of the astral experience goes along the lines of mitigating emotional distress and nervousness, and health conditions such as insomnia.

Some modern health practitioners are today using the valerian root alongside other herbs that have sedating properties, the purpose being to enhance the experience of astral projection. Such herbs include the lemon balm, whose botanical name is Melissa Officinalis, and hops that is scientifically referred to as humulus lupulus.

Nevertheless, the combination of these herbs is sometimes used simply to solve issues of sleep deprivation.

The Mugwort herb or Artemisia Vulgaris

The Mugwort, which is also called the felon or sailor's tobacco, is a perennial plant, and it belongs to the family of the Compositae.

An interesting fact about this plant is that it was the basic beer-making ingredient prior to the discovery of hops. You may find this herb also referred to as the chrysanthemum weed or moxa.

One of the most significant properties of this herb is enhancement of blood circulation as the blood enters the uterus and the pelvic region. Effectively, it causes stimulation of menstruation. It is actually seen as playing the role of an emmenagogue, a medicinal substance purposely meant to stimulate the flow of menstrual blood.

With regard to astral projection, some people have reported having out of body experiences, while others have reported having dreams of a prophetic nature, after enjoying having puffs of the mugwort the way people smoke tobacco.

The Heimia Salicifolia Herb

The Heimia Salicifolia, otherwise referred to as narrow leaf heimia or sun opener, is a shrub whose branches develop closely in a dense manner. It belongs to the family of flowering shrubs known as loosestrife.

Shamans value this herb because they credit it with enhancing their capacity to recall events; even those that occurred way back in the past.

The kind of memory enhancement the heimia salicifolia does is not at the usual level; this one is higher. For example, some shamans have professed having been aided by the herb to remember events that happened before their own births. They also praise the herb's capacity to enhance one's experience in astral projection.

The Wild Asparagus or Asparagus Racemosus

The wild asparagus also goes by the term 'flying herb,' and although some people call it the Chinese asparagus, the herb is actually said to have originated within the Mediterranean region.

This herb that thrives in mountainous terrain, has always been popular within the Chinese as well as Korean cultures, as a potent medicinal herb.

The part of this herb used for medicinal purposes is the root, which is also credited with capacity to aid astral projection. It is also an herb shamans rely on for their spiritual growth and development.

In fact, the reason the herb is referred to as 'flying herb' is that it enables the individual to traverse the universe in flight mode, in the process experiencing dreams in their lucid form.

Besides shamans, other spiritual individuals who make use of the Heimia Salicifolia Herb to enhance their experiences include yogis and monks. They find the herb to have strong capacity to open the 'anahata,' which is essentially the heart chakra.

It is worth noting that the heart chakra is the energy center responsible for emotional balance; and if it is in good balance you do not experience anxiety. Without anxiety, you are in a good position to experience your journey to the astral world; and hence the reason shamans attached a lot of importance to the flying herb.

Anther community that attached exceptional importance to the wild asparagus is that of the Taoists. They credited the Chinese asparagus with enhancing people's potential to reach mental levels beyond the mundane.

The Rosemary Herb or Rosmarinus officinalis

The Rosemary herb is also referred to as the remembrance herb. This aromatic herb is perennial, and it is known to thrive to an age of 18yrs.

The reasons shamans and other spiritual people value it is not only its capacity as a stress reliever, but also its efficacy in enhancing mental lucidity. They also found that the herb improved their memory.

The Bitter Grass or Calea Zacatechichi

The bitter grass herb, also referred to as 'dream herb,' originated in Central America as well as areas of Mexico.

The herb is credited with enhancing lucidity when dreaming, and also the experience in astral projection.

Other attributes credited to bitter grass include its capacity to enhance a person's dream frequency and capacity to recall the dreams; enhancement of one's reaction speed and mental clearness; as well as its effect of increasing an individual's peace.

The Maidenhair Tree or Ginkgo Biloba

The maidenhair tree is a medicinal plant whose use dates centuries ago. For example, the Chinese have been using the Ginkgo Biloba for more than a thousand two hundred years.

The reason this herb is great at enhancing the astral projection experience is that it has capacity to enhance the flow of blood within the brain. This, in turn, improves your mental clarity.

Ginkgo Biloba is also credited with enhancing memory, something that is important if your astral projection is to be helpful in your day-to-day life.

This plant is also credited with treating mental health conditions like depression and Attention Deficiency Hyperactivity Disorder. The capacity this plant has to enhance your mental function will contribute to enhancing your astral projection experience.

Thyme or Thymus Vulgaris

Thyme that is part of the family of mints is found in very many species. Though popular for its culinary value, with ancient Romans using it to flavor their alcoholic drinks as well as cheese, it is also valued for its capacity to enhance the respiratory function.

Also, through its capacity to improve the nervous function, it ends up enhancing your ability to experience astral projection. In fact, this herb is directly linked to clarity of the mind and enhancement of psychic comprehension.

Consciousness & Shamanism

Generally, it is the belief of Native Americans that the universe is a unitary world whose existence is cohesive, and which contains a soul; and that everything that exists in this sphere not only has some life, but also consciousness.

Even things like minerals that existed within earth the mother are considered to be living things. In fact, the formation of iron, bronze and other minerals, including the stage of smelting, is considered a spiritual process of purification; and sometimes shamans would partake in meditation and other actions of a cultic nature.

It is important to note that according to Buddhism, the physical and spiritual bodies are intertwined, and you cannot separate one from the other. This essentially means that a person comprises a body and a soul that merge to form the human being.

Even then, the soul part of the person is finer and is not tangible like the body component. This makes it possible for the soul to exist in the person's dream while not being seen or felt in the body.

There is, nevertheless, another time when the soul can be detected. A shaman can discern the existence of the soul during his/her travels.

As far as relationships among individuals are concerned, ethnologists find them mystical; unique experiences that connect every person to others within his/her community. This can be understood to mean that whatever an individual goes through has some impact on the mood or health of the group to which he/she belongs.

Shamans believe in deities; taking many of them to be ordinarily superior to human beings. These deities are considered to have much more knowledge and even power, than regular human beings.

Nevertheless, there is a way deities are able to align their superior knowledge with that of human beings, and the people who are involved have traditionally formed high-caliber cultures.

How to Work with Consciousness

When shamans practiced, every individual would reach his unique level of consciousness, with a given degree of spiritual power that is referred to as 'mana.' This power was responsible for determining the intrinsic value an individual or an animal had.

A person with tremendous spiritual power would essentially possess great psychic energy. For individuals who have had sufficient practice, for example, in astral projection, their skills would complement their significant psychic power, and they would be successful in entering diverse levels of consciousness.

This spiritual endowment would help these shamans succeed in their undertakings, not only those involving healing and cultural rites, but also those that helped in everyday survival, like hunting.

Suffice it to say, abundance in psychic energy is a fundamental part of a shaman's life, his/her life as a religious being, as well as his/her social life. A shaman is, therefore, able to experience different life phases as a natural way of life.

The techniques used in shamanism to systematically transform a person from one state of consciousness to another are considered the most ancient of all techniques. It needs to be understood that shamanism has been in practice since the period from around 30,000 to 40,000 B.C.

Though different communities have had their different ways of describing their astral techniques, a fundamental link has been found to exist in all of them. One expert who has documented comprehensive descriptions pertaining to shamanism is Mircea Eliade, whose specialty is the history of religion.

In his explanation regarding the way someone becomes a shaman, Eliade indicates that one is considered suitable to become a shaman after it has been noted the person has special capabilities as far as matters of consciousness are concerned.

Such a person is found to be contemplative, and a dreamer who experiences visions of a prophetic nature. This is also the kind of individual who cherishes solitude; and who is sometimes oddly reclusive.

In preparing a person to become a shaman, he/she is taken through some training, with the intention of reinforcing those special qualities already observed. During this training, the individual is physically isolated from everyone else; and he ceases to partake of everyday activities.

There are also cases when an individual succeeds to become a shaman by experiencing some physical ailment.

Shamanic Experiences

When a shaman is going through transitions to varying states of consciousness, he/she experiences some intensity and power that give him insight into gloomy or unpleasant matters. The varying levels of intensity and power are also enabling the person to acquire some kind of magical control.

Still, there are times when the shaman might find it necessary to increase his/her level of control; and in such times it is usual to make use of some form of intoxicants, and then proceed to dance in an atmosphere of darkness. It is also normal for the shaman, at such times, to use other methods he/she deems appropriate, to enter into a trance.

Where shamanism is practiced, it plays an important role in the society; often offering much-needed prophesies. At other times, the techniques of shamanism are employed alongside treatments of psychosomatic issues. This means shamans may also depended upon to assist in the treatment of people who have mental and psychological issues.

In shamanism, it is believed that once you succeed in detaching yourself from your normal or ordinary awareness, you find yourself elevated to other consciousness levels. Once in a different level of consciousness, you have access to information you would not otherwise reach. You also have better insights to matters of communal benefit to people around you, which ordinarily you would not have.

Once on an elevated level of consciousness, you are not only more imaginative, but you also gain information in a manner that is symbolic. You also have more clarity on significant matters.

In many traditions that appreciate shamanism, people who are able to reach higher levels of consciousness have a better understanding of the dreams they experience, than those who do not. It is believed that a person's soul is involved when it comes to the experiences he/she has in the higher levels of consciousness.

Dreams that involve individuals are ordinarily considered to be small, while those that involve a community as a whole are considered big. The big dreams are of benefit to the entire community, and they serve to improve matters of a societal and cultural value.

Individuals with potential to become shamans normally have dreams of value to the community at large; big dreams. According to ancient traditions, big dreams normally come from shamans or medicine men, or even priests.

Wholesome Healing of Body & Soul

Ancient communities have been found by scholars like Lévi-Strauss to have possessed superior skills with regard to the treatment of illnesses of a psychosomatic and psychic nature. This is because the transformation from ordinary level of consciousness to higher ones does not exist in modern medicine.

This capacity to reach higher consciousness levels combines with the belief people have in spirits to help provide guidance regarding which healing methods are appropriate for individual cases.

Shamans have, for example, been able to treat people deemed to be mentally unstable; or to be possessed. The shaman in charge enters a different consciousness level and travels to the higher world where spirits dwell, and manages to retrieve the sanity or 'soul' the affected individual is considered to have lost. In short, shamans have powers of a magical nature, which modern doctors are not known to have.

The entire process might appear dramatic to the ordinary observer, but people who appeared to have lost their souls have been known to return to normal after interventions from shamans.

How to Tell a Person is possessed

There are different ways a possessed person betrays his/her state. One of them is a person having his/her identity lost; which means the behavior the person is manifesting is that of a different person.

You may even the person's look to be different, even as he/she walks and speaks differently. In short, a person who is possessed can adopt an entirely different set of behaviors. His / Her character dramatically changes, and even his/her physical body movements are transformed.

While some people will have lost consciousness as they manifest this altered behavior, some are somewhat aware of their actions. The explanation here is that this person who is aware of what he/she is doing and saying will be doing so as a representative of a certain spirit that will have invaded his/her being. So it is not the person you know talking or acting at this time; but the spirit inside him/her.

After such an experience, the affected person does not recall any of the things you attribute to him/her.

It is said that being possessed is not always a health condition. Some people are said to have capacity to consciously provoke such possession.

The reason a person may wish to assume a possessed state is so that he/she can serve as a medium; and to have capacity to connect with higher beings. If you succeed in assuming the role of a medium, what you say is the voice of the spirit you will have connected with.

How to Treat Possession

Once a person is deemed to be possessed and there is need to bring him/her back to normal existence, the process used is known as exorcism. Essentially, exorcism entails the act of driving away evil spirits.

In modern civilizations, exorcism is acknowledged, and is particularly known to have played a big role in the Western culture. The church is known to have used exorcism for many years; official records putting the end of this practice to be around the 1700s.

It is important to note that although a person possessed normally has the spirit of an ancestor or some god, sometimes the spirit could be from a sorcerer, animal, or even a demon.

Role of an Exorcist

An apt definition of an exorcist is a person who acts on behalf of a higher power with regard to getting rid of spirits, and is able to convince people that his connection to such great powers is genuine.

The starting point for an exorcist is to influence the spirit or put pressure on it, with a view to having it reveal itself. Thereafter, he embarks on trying to drive out that spirit. The success of an exorcist in driving out a spirit lies in his capacity to negotiate with it, although he/she sometimes seeks help from friendly spirits.

Spirits often ready to assist exorcists include the gods that traditionally control nature, and for Christians it can be those acknowledged biblically.

As the exorcism takes place, the person who is possessed is put into a state of trance; sometimes through a process of intense dancing, and other times through mental suggestions. Whatever process is used to get the person into a trance depends on the setting.

It is easy to know when the person has entered the state of trance, because that state is underlined by fierce tremors and convulsions; and other movements of the body like twitches.

The person can also break into an emotional outburst that is ordinarily violent in nature, a development understood to be a manifestation of demons.

In order for this individual to go over that violent phase, it is considered necessary to dramatically carry out negotiations, and once this attempt has been successful the person collapses into limpness.

Modern doctors including psychiatrists have acknowledged the positive role exorcism plays in treating cases of psychic and even psychosomatic nature. Even ethnologists appreciate the roles exorcists play.

Within the Christian faith, an Austrian priest known as Johan J. Gassner is said to have been the last church leader to treat possessed people through exorcism. This parish priest lived from 1727 to 1779.

Feelings of True Self-identity

It is important to understand that just as individual plants are identifiable through their unique characteristics, so is the identification of every individual. Every person is unique. That is the nature of God's creations.

Also, just as every species of plant has a climate that suits it, so has every person an environment suitable for him/her.

Polar bears, for example, live comfortably in the arctic region, but they would very likely not survive anywhere along the Equator. Likewise, the palm trees that grow tall within the hot desert climate of Southern California would not survive in the cold desert of Siberia.

In short, God had a purpose for making every living thing the way it is, and placing it where on earth it is. For that reason, it is hoped that every living being appreciates its unique attributes, size and design.

Unfortunately, human beings do not always live up to this hope. Many keep comparing themselves with others they know, thinking they would be happier if they were like them. The best way for people to contribute optimally to the wellbeing of the universe and everything in it is to appreciate your unique qualities, and to make use of these abilities to the optimum. It is also the simplest way to live a fulfilled life.

Human Beings as Seeds

Since God gave you your own uniqueness as part of the human race, you should consider yourself a seed, which God made in a special way and placed it in its unique environment.

Your Creator understood the environmental conditions you are able to survive in; and once you understand this you will begin to look for what it is you can accomplish under your circumstances; instead of spending time trying to change your environment.

In other words, you are complete the way you are, and in a position to accomplish great things wherever you are.

The best advice you could take is to cease looking for things, people or conditions to complete you. When you go looking for such things, you are essentially seeking a different identity; one that is not yours and hence false.

Your true identity is the individual you are with whatever God has bestowed upon you, and within the environment He has allowed you to be in. Once you acknowledge this fact you begin to appreciate your value, since every person's value is as inherent as the value of a seed.

The worth of a seed is not dependent on how well it can survive a cold or hot season, how high its plant is capable of growing, or any other variant. Rather, its value is that which the farmer knows of it even before proceeding to plant it.

A farmer leaves other seeds available in the market and only chooses one to go and plant because that is the one he/she has faith in; belief that it has what it takes to give him/her benefit. Likewise, your worth is not pegged on what other people think of your potential; rather it is inbuilt and only waiting to manifest when time is suitable.

It is important to note that although human beings exist in their mortal bodies, every person's spirit has been in existence even prior to the individual being born. The same thing applies to a person's potential.

In short, there are different spheres of existence before physical birth and after death; the one after physical death being eternal existence.

BOOK 16

AMERICAN EDIBLE WILD PLANTS

CHAPTER 1

TIPS & NEED FOR ETHICAL FORAGING

For several centuries, people survived through hunting and foraging; the reason they were said to be hunters and gatherers. The hunting part was not only scary sometimes; it was also a big challenge. For this reason, foraging made survival much easier because even without meat, people could live on plant food that was found to be nutritious.

Purpose of Foraging

It needs to be remembered that a lot of plant food also has a medicinal element. Also considering that foraging is a relatively safe undertaking, children and their mothers could participate and hence make work easier.

That is why even just a century ago North American women would pick chickweed, which is very prolific and hardy, and use it at home during winter when it was generally difficult to find newly picked vegetables in stores. Cooks of the Victorian era were confident they could always find fresh chickweed in winter, meaning their meals were never short of fresh vegetables.

Besides, this is one of the most nutritious plants available in the wild. Not only does it contain Vitamins A, C, D and B6 plus B12, but it also has minerals that include magnesium and phosphorus. Chickweed would be served even as a salad; and people would enjoy the crispiness of its leaves that also happened to be tender.

It is worth reminding people of the role foraging played in those olden days, because then they might reflect before destroying the plants that exist today without being purposefully cultivated. A plant like the chickweed is today viewed by many as a weed whose existence is inconsequential, and hence destroyed without a second thought.

By reading informational books pertaining to the importance of herbs and role of foraging, people might choose to regain the art of plant identification and careful harvesting of wild plants for culinary and other uses.

Actually, it is the caring part that is most pertinent, considering that today several luxurious restaurants have begun to embrace wild foods mostly foraged from their natural habitats.

Generally also, there seems to be a renewed interest in foods that have previously been shunned as weeds without much use, with people rediscovering that these plants are not only highly palatable, but also highly nutritious and medicinal.

There is also the realization that foraging comes with some unique satisfaction; a high that one feels after succeeding in gathering sufficient leaves, berries or even roots needed either for food or medicine.

Foraging comes with an added health benefit that may sometimes go unacknowledged, and that is the calming effect one experiences while on the mission. Foraging is very beneficial to the person doing it, especially when one takes it as a hobby.

After a long day of work, for instance, walking through some natural habitat and being able to identify nature's own treasure serves as a welcome antidote.

For the sake of carrying on the practice of safe foraging, it is advisable that people who read and learn about safe and medicinal plants share that information with the younger generation.

In fact, it is recommended that you take the children around you to the wild when going foraging, so you can curtail the addictive culture of TV, mobile phones and video games, which is becoming more and more entrenched among the young.

For those children who may find it punitive to leave their phones behind, take advantage of that attachment and let the children try to search specific weeds online. It should serve to promote their skills in correctly identifying edible plants. Help the children identify plants not only by their descriptions, but also through their photos.

It is important to point out that the term 'foraging' does not only applicable to the search for plants in forested areas or in rural set ups. It is also applicable when you go looking for plants alongside roads, paths or playgrounds; as long as these plants are growing naturally and nobody is tending to them.

One important message you need to always pass to everyone learning to forage is that it is paramount that you do not exhaust any one area of its plants. The reason is not only consideration for the next person seeking to find some foodstuff, but the need to have parent plants and seeds for continuity of the species.

Besides, there are also animals that rely on these plants as their natural source of food. In fact, it is advisable to pick the leaves, twigs or fruits you need, as opposed to pulling out plants and uprooting them totally.

It is also important to keep in mind that as you go foraging, the intention is to gain something you need but not to destroy what you do not need. This means that whether a plant is edible or not, medicinal or not, it has an important role to play in its natural habitat.

You should, therefore, disabuse the notion that it is fine to tread on plants you do not need as you make your way through bushes to find the plants you are interested in. After all, you are not the only being depending on the growths for health and survival.

To qualify to call yourself a forager, you must have a good understanding of nature and how best to preserve the environment. True foragers are not only skilled at plant identification; they are also skilled at preparing wild plants for food and medicine.

For example, they understand the parts of plants they need to harvest for particular medications; meaning they do not unnecessarily harvest plant parts they do not need when they are interested in extracting material for medicinal use.

Foraging with care and skill strengthens the relationship foragers have with the environment, and it ensures the ecosystem remains stable.

The danger that should draw your attention is that of ill informed people who venture into the wild and are overly zealous in their plant harvesting. When you encounter such people, you would do some good by advising them on the danger of overharvesting; and give them tips on how best to safeguard the area even as they find the plants they want.

The bottom line is that foraging can continue to be helpful to people and the environment as long as it is done with care. In fact, foraging is healthy as long as nature's universal rule is followed – keeping in mind that just as in math, there is a limit to every function.

How to Entrench Ethical Foraging

Even without curtailing people's fun and excitement in foraging, and even without robbing them of the therapeutic benefit of the practice, care can be taken to forage responsibly.

That way, people enjoy the benefits derived from the use of plants, and the environment thrives to provide more benefit on a continued basis. Here next are things you can do to help you carry out your foraging missions in an ethical manner.

Studying the Area

Before anyone can embark on foraging, they need to know the flora prevalent in the particular area. Some of the available plants may be few in species and number, while others may be abundant both in species and plant population.

Such abundance or scarcity should tell you if a plant is at risk of extinction; and hence the need to be careful how you handle it.

Considering as a knowledgeable forager you want to remain ethical, you need to make sure you spare any plants that are rare in the area, and forage only those present in abundance.

Often you do not need to wait until you can do a physical check for you to know the plant species in danger of being depleted in a given region. Normally regional libraries have crucial information on local flora, and you can check in to learn the specifics.

Besides learning about rarity or prolificacy of individual plant species, you also need to be informed about the conditions under which individual plants thrive. This includes learning how the plants behave in different seasons and not only under specific weather conditions. This information is paramount in guiding your behavior as you undertake your foraging events.

For example, you will know when it is destructive to pluck flowers from certain plants, and when it is fine to do so. It would be unfortunate if you were to pluck flowers off a plant just when they were about to produce berries; and probably you just wanted the flowers to make your living room beautiful.

Note that if you make such a mistake, you deny yourself and other people interested in foraging an opportunity to enjoy berries from those plants.

Although this explanation regarding not depriving plants of an opportunity to bear fruit is important, there may be several more reasons why you should spare certain plants as you forage.

For this reason, you need to talk to local residents regarding their environment and the things they hold dear as far as the wilds around them are concerned. If possible, it is a good idea to seek the views of different foragers and hunters, and consult the fishing community if there is a fishing area in the neighborhood.

The basic point is that there is need to have a word with all stakeholders in a given region before embarking on a foraging mission; because you get to have better insights pertaining to the region's flora and fauna, and even their inter-dependence.

Creating a Plan

It is important to draw a plan before you can embark on any foraging mission. Many successful missions start off with a plan, and foraging should not be any exception.

For starters, make a point of learning the location where you intend to do the foraging. Another important thing is being clear about what you want to find; as in the specific herb you will be searching.

It is important that once you are certain about the plant you want and its general location, you make a point of sticking to your plan.

It may appear a little bit too strict to insist you do not get diverted from your plan, especially considering the wild is normally rich in plant varieties; but much as it is normal to be interested in plants new to you, the best foraging etiquette entails you taking pictures of those plants. You can proceed to document any other plants that draw your attention, for the purpose of following on them later.

Accurate Plant & Area Identification

People need to be aware that many regions usually have field guides, and so if you can identify a guide near you, it is advisable to utilize his/her guidance for purposes of foraging.

Guided foraging is great at minimizing, if not eliminating, misidentification of specific plant species. It is also crucial at ensuring you do not harvest a plant that falls under the endangered species.

The importance of accurate identification of plant species is very important, and so before proceeding on your foraging mission, it is crucial that you have the skills to pinpoint the exact plant you want.

Note that precision in identifying plants should extend even to the smaller plant species like the mushrooms. In order to eliminate errors in plant identification, you need to have more than a single way of identifying a plant.

For example, instead of restricting yourself to identifying a particular plant through the look of its leaves, learn what the plant stem and its leaves look like. In addition, make a point of learning when the particular plant blooms.

With such knowledge, it is very unlikely you are going to misidentify the plant you want. Other attributes that may help you identify individual plant species with accuracy include the fragrance of that plant, its life cycle, the look of its fruits, the color of its leaves, the plant's location, the look of the plant's branches and its bark, the conditions of the soil the plant in which the plant thrives, as well as the plant's spore prints.

People need to keep in mind the importance of choosing appropriately what plants to harvest, and not just the area to go for foraging.

If the plants available literally line the highway, or if they are within some industrial location, it is best to leave them alone. Leave herbs alone also if those available are markings around particular properties.

The most pertinent reason for such warning is that these are among the most polluted areas; which means if you forage in such places you risk ending up with contaminated plants.

Note that plants meant for culinary or medicinal purposes should always be suitable for consumption. Without a doubt, if people consume plants that have been exposed to pollutants, they will be consuming toxic substances albeit in an indirect manner.

Even as you keep in mind those areas risky for foraging, you need to know those areas most suitable for the practice. The first quality you need to look for is detachment from habited land. Areas where there is little or no human activity are best for foraging, because the area is unlikely to have been interfered with.

This means the range of plant species in the area is likely to be large, plants are likely to be prolific in terms of the fruits they bear, and they are likely to be healthy and free from pollutants. In other words, natural habitats have the cleanest and safest herbs for human consumption.

Remain Conservative with your Foraging

When it is time to harvest herbs, make a point of harvesting just what is necessary; but not what is available. You will be reasonable to remember you are not the only one in need of natural herbs, whether for your kitchen or your medical emergency kit.

In the spirit of willingness to share, spare as many medicinal herbs as you can. In regions where people forage without consideration for others or the future, important herbs get depleted very fast. At the end of the day, everyone is no longer able to reap the benefits that the wild offers.

It is always good to remember the herb harvesting rule of thumb, which is that you should avoid harvesting over a third of a given patch of herbs. Practically, you need to leave your target herb alone if in the region you are surveying there is only one patch of that herb. However, if you find three such patches, it will be fine to harvest the herbs from one of them.

As an ethical forager, you are expected to adhere to this convention because you understand the importance of maintaining a good natural balance. It is also assumed you understand the need to be considerate of all other living things, inclusive of your fellow people.

Some people might be afraid that if you do not harvest the first patch of herbs you find you may never manage to retrace it later, but there is a way you can avoid such a complication. You can ensure you will be able to find your way back to the target patch of herb by marking the particular spot. Making such an effort is preferable to harvesting an herb that is among the endangered species.

Safeguard the Landscape

Foragers are always advised to try as much as they can to leave the landscape unaltered. One of the things that can lead to altered landscapes is excessive herb harvesting, and poor harvesting techniques.

Generally, natural landscape is beautiful, and you can tell a piece of area has been badly handled if the landscape does not reflect its natural beauty. Basically, what is being asked of you as a responsible forager is to avoid ransacking and pillaging an herbal habitat in the name of foraging.

Another telltale sign the wilds have been badly handled is visible litter. Even if the local authorities have not put up signs against making the place dirty, you are expected to be reasonable enough to handle your garbage in a decent manner.

After all, anyone who cherishes the wellbeing of the human race and all other living things that make people's lives worthwhile should ensure plants grow in a clean area the same way people like living in a clean environment.

As a forager who cares for the environment, you can take it upon yourself to collect any litter you find in the wrong places, even when you are not responsible for making the place dirty. In fact, foragers are advised to take a spare bag with them when they go herb harvesting just in case they find garbage that they need to collect.

On the overall, you should do everything you can to improve the plant habitat, and also avoid everything that would threaten that same environment and the living things within it. The behaviors to avoid include unnecessary harvesting of tree branches; unwarranted cutting down of trees; carelessly causing disturbance to bird nests; and the habit of recklessly driving off-road.

Besides being personally careful to safeguard the integrity of forests, shrubberies and other natural habitats, you would do nature a lot of good if you made a point of reporting any destruction you notice in the wild. Reporting to the local authorities or any other relevant bodies any conditions you find unfit for plants to thrive can ensure the problem is solved before it can exacerbate to levels difficult to reverse.

Adhere to Legal Stipulations

Before you begin seeking the best places to forage or the best herbs to utilize for your herbal practice, you need to learn the rules that need to be followed by foragers. This means that much as foraging ethically is important, it is even more important to forage within the law.

Local regulations as well as guidelines are also critical, and you should prioritize learning them. Adherence to the stipulations set by local authorities is crucial to your success.

Learn the permits required for you to forage within the law, and make a point of acquiring them. This is crucial so that you can avoid committing trespass, or breaking other laws set by your state or other local agents. Potential foragers need to keep in mind that ignorance, according to legal authorities, is not an acceptable excuse.

Besides avoiding the risk of committing trespass on government land, you also need to take care not to trespass on privately owned properties. This means if land is not your own, it is best that you seek the necessary permission from the owner.

All in all, you are bound to enjoy your foraging exercise and to succeed in finding what you are interested in, if you carry out your functions in harmony with the community around you.

After all, as is the belief in shamanism, everything and everyone in the universe has to exist in harmony for all to succeed.

In case you are entirely new to a region you are interested in, or it is the first time you are considering foraging in the area, it would be helpful to consult the area residents. Have conversations with those knowledgeable, and seek the permissions necessary and acquire the necessary documentation. In short, you need to go through the steps necessary in the process to legally becoming a forager.

Another factor any new forager has to consider if he/she is to succeed in carrying out safe and worthwhile foraging involves the hunting seasons in the local area. It is crucial that you understand them alongside the hunting schedules put in place by the relevant authorities.

Failure to do so would put you at the risk of being fined, and to cause disharmony with parties interested in safeguarding the local habitat.

After all is said and done, people need to appreciate that nature has enough for everyone in the universe; and when some seem to be lacking it is because there is sometimes poor management of resources.

It is, therefore, imperative that every person does whatever it takes to safeguard the universe and every part of nature in existence. For a forager interested in doing things right for the welfare of mankind and the universe at large, you need to ensure your foraging trips are well planned, and when the foraging process begins it is carried out ethically and with appropriate restraint.

Prepare Appropriately

The preparation explained here involves ensuring the entire foraging mission goes on successfully, and that you do not fail to harvest any herb you need because of lack of equipment or carrying containers.

Wear Appropriate Clothing

Just as it is important to plan of action before venturing into any foraging zone, it is crucial that make the necessary preparations before starting your journey outdoors. Preparation in this context involves having the right form of clothing; and also equipping yourself with the right tools.

First of all, it is crucial that you wear comfortable clothing when going out to forage, to ensure ease of movement. If moving about is easy for you, it follows that you are unlikely to have some parts of your garment getting entangled with the vegetation.

At the same time, you are not expected to wear the kind of clothes you take to some high-end laundry for cleaning. In short, some old clothes will do. This is because you cannot rule out some thorn sticking out of some shrub giving your clothing some tears and rips.

It also helps to be practical when considering the clothing to wear or pack, and this includes acknowledging the possibility of rain falling. In this regard, it is a good idea to take with you a raincoat, or a simple jacket that is waterproof.

Carry Appropriate Equipment

Among the basic equipment you need to carry with you is a map, herb-gathering receptacles, lighting and cooking equipment, and any other piece of equipment personal to you.

You need to take with you a map of the local area, and the reason for this is to be certain you will be able to find your way around and back without a hitch.

Note that losing your way while foraging might cause you to stray into protected territory, or even onto privately owned property. Besides, you may get lost for so many hours that it gets dark before you find your way back, and if this happens there would be the risk of you treading on herbs and damaging them.

As for herb-gathering receptacles, every one of them should be suitable to the part of the plant you intend to harvest. For example, if your intention is to harvest some berries, tiny fruits or mushrooms, tiny plastic boxes would be suitable.

It is also important to know that you can substitute plastic containers with Tupperware or some other containers with lids. The reason these can be substituted without any inconvenience is that they can safely hold herb delicate herbs or herb products without them getting crushed.

For example, if you harvest grapes, berries or apricots and put them in a covered container, they will be safe by the time you get home even if you travel a long distance through the woods. In short, herb items that can be easily smashed should not be put in a shopping bag. Covered containers are best for such items.

Other items that are safe being carried in Tupperware include fresh flowers, and thorny herbs such as milk thistle or prickly pear. The best thing in putting thorny items in such containers is that the material these containers are made of cannot be torn by the thorns.

In case you intend to harvest roots or big fruits, you may need to carry some medium-sized baskets.

Note it is not always you need to buy containers specifically for your foraging missions. When you want forage big herbs in big quantities, you can use the common shopping bags made of plastic. These ones are particularly suitable for herbs like the mallow and purslane, and others like the mustard.

These plastic bags are also appropriate for large-sized fruits such as apples and lemons, and nuts like the walnuts.

Alternatively, you can carry those small bags meant for sandwiches if you are going out to forage seeds, pine nuts and such other tiny plant materials. Anything too small to hold in a shopping bag can go into a sandwich bag.

It is also advisable to carry freezer bags in instances when you are planning to forage for plantain or such other plants that you can easily lose through a shopping bag's tiny holes.

Generally as a frequent forager, you need to have some containers of varying sizes, preferably plastic because they are rust-free, so that you can pick the most appropriate as need be.

A torch is always a necessity even if it is daytime when you leave for the wild. This is because things do not always go according to plan. It has been noted that sometimes, especially in autumn when thriving herbs are in plenty, foragers get carried away in their mission and often lose count of time. As such, many of them end up exiting the wild in darkness.

It is also advisable to take a mobile phone with you even if your intention is not to keep engaging with the outside world as you carry out your herb harvesting. The importance of being able to communicate is that if you found yourself in an emergency situation you would have no problem calling for assistance.

Some cooking equipment, such as a camping stove, is necessary if you think your foraging is going to take a whole day. In situations where you are certain you will need to sit somewhere and have a meal; it is a good idea to pack some mats and other odds and ends relevant to this kind of setting.

And even if you do not plan on having a full meal out in the wild, you should remember to carry a small carrier bag for your drinking water, snacks, probably some first aid items, and any other small items personal to you.

Carry Appropriate Herb-Picking Tools

Obviously, your foraging mission cannot begin unless you have tools suitable to harvest the herbs you need. Such are the kind of tools that while getting you the part of plant you wan will not harm the mother plant. You need to remember that the basis of herb growing continuity lies in foragers carrying out their harvesting in a non-destructive manner.

It is also important that the tools you use be safe for you too; you should avoid using tools or equipment that can easily hurt your hands or cause them blistering. At the same time, it is important that you equip yourself with protective material for the purpose of safeguarding your hands from thorns and such other plant parts that can prick you.

Among the handiest tools are scissors, hand gloves, mitts, hand trowels and such others. You can actually acquire a forager's kit in which to put all these tiny but very important tools.

The reason you need some scissors is that some of the part of the plant you want require severing, and if you use your hands it may be a struggle. Other times, like when you need a twig, getting it off the plant stem may not be difficult, but you may risk peeling off the bark of the plant.

For some plants, peeling off the bark, or even part of it, may retard the development of the plant. Also, if you struggle a lot trying to break a twig, you may break the entire plant especially if the stem is fragile.

There are also those plant parts that you risk crushing if you use hands to pick them; like some berries that develop as a batch.

Something else that makes a pair of scissors a handy tool is that if the herb you are harvesting is prickly, you could get hurt using your bare hands.

In case you are interested in the stem of the plant, you can use the pair of scissors to sever the stem from some place close to the base, leaving the root safe with potential to shoot afresh.

Something else you need to pack in your tool bag is a pair of gardening gloves. These ones are meant to protect your hands as you forage for herbs. Not only do the gloves protect you from being stung by thorns, but they also protect you from the stings of plants like the stinging nettle.

For the sake of protecting yourself from plants from which gloves cannot effectively protect you, it is advisable to also equip yourself with some sturdy mitts like those of hard plastic. Such mitts come in handy when you want to harvest plant parts that are prickly; like prickly pears whose mother plant belongs to the family of cactuses.

You would also be saving yourself unnecessary costs when you use mitts instead of gloves for prickly herbs, considering if you used gloves you would have to discard them once the mission is over. The reason you cannot reuse the gloves is that the spikes prick the gloves and stubbornly stick there. This does not happen to mitts.

In case you discover another tool that is helpful in foraging, make a point of adding it to your list of foraging tools to pack for the mission.

BOOK 17

HERBAL MEDICINES & PLANT REMEDIES. - VOLUME 1

1. ALFALFA

SCIENTIFIC NAME: MEDICAGO ATIVA

COMMON NAME: LUCERNE AND BUFFALO HERB

FAMILY: FABACEAE

ORIGIN: BROUGHT TO AMERICA FROM ASIA.

USE AND BENEFITS:

In Asia, alfalfa dates back thousands of years, yet it arrived in North America only in the 1860s. This deep-rooted shrub may also be found in the United States from Virginia to Maine, as well as west to the Pacific coastlines. For the treatment of urinary tract and prostate problems, this plant includes seeds, sprouts, and leaves. Relieves menopausal symptoms while also boosting metabolism and lowering cholesterol.

2. MINT

SCIENTIFIC NAME: MENTHA

COMMON NAME: MINT

FAMILY: LAMIACEAE

ORIGIN: MEDITERRANEAN REGION AND ASIA

USE AND BENEFITS:

It's also been used for indigestion, respiratory issues, heartburn, common cold, flu, allergies, headaches, and as a light sedative for a long time. It's been used to cure itching, small burns, acne and skin irritations on the outside. The stems and leaves were utilized by the Cherokee to treat high blood pressure.

3. Horsemint

Scientific name: Mentha Longifolia
Common names: bergamot, horsemint, bee balm
Family: Mint family
Origin: Asia and Europe

Use and Benefits: It has traditionally been prized for its antibacterial powers and digestive effects. Teas and tonics made from the leaves and flowering stalks have been used to alleviate fever, headaches, and inflammation.

4. Wormwood

Scientific name: Artemisia absinthium
Common names: green ginger and absinthe
Family: Asteraceae
Origin: Eurasia and northern Africa's temperate zones are home to this species.

Use and Benefits: The leaves and flower tips were collected and dried for use in tonics for stomach pain, indigestion, labor pain, heartburn, and lack of appetite. Bronchitis was reportedly treated using a tea made from boiling leaves of a native variety of wormwood by the Yokia Indians.

5. Dogwood

Scientific name: Cornus florida
Common names: boxwood, American dogwood, cornelian tree, budwood, green ozier, and flowering dogwood
Family: Cornaceae
Origin: native to the United States

Use and Benefits: Internally, it was mostly used to cure fever, malaria, colds, pneumonia, and diarrhea and also to aid digestion and appetite. Poultices were used externally to treat ulcers and wounds. Poultices were also manufactured, which were used to treat wounds and other skin conditions. The Arikara blended the bark with bearberry to produce holy tobacco, while the Menominee used it in enemas. During the Civil War, it was commonly used in the South to treat chronic diarrhea and malarial fever.

6. Damiana

Scientific name: Turnera diffusa
Common names: damiana
Family: Passifloraceae
Origin: Southwest Texas, Central America, southern California, South

Use and Benefits: America, Mexico, and the Caribbean are all home to this species. It's long been thought to stimulate libido, and it's still used as an aphrodisiac today. It has also been used to treat asthma, depression, impotence, menstruation issues, anxiety, nervousness, and constipation, as well as to enhance energy and improve digestion.

7. Ginger Root

Scientific name: Zingiber Officinale
Common names: Ginger
Family: Zingiberaceae
Origin: Southeast Asia's Maritime Region

Use and Benefits: It's been used for a long time to treat digestive issues and nausea, including motion sickness, bloating, heartburn, flatulence, and gastrointestinal issues. Colic, irritable bowel syndrome, lack of appetite, chills, colds, flu, menstrual cramps, stomach cramps, poor circulation, fever, headaches, toothache, cough, and bronchitis are all conditions for which it is used. It has been used for joint disorders, arthritis, rheumatism, and tendonitis as well as being a powerful anti-inflammatory plant. It is also said to help decrease cholesterol and blood pressure, as well as prevent internal blood clots.

8. Dogbane

Scientific name: Apocynum cannabinum
Common names: Indian hemp & hemp dogbane
Family: Apocynaceae
Origin: North American native

Use and Benefits: It is used to treat fever and diarrhea in herbal medicine. Although the plant's toxins may produce catharsis and nausea, it has reportedly been utilized to lower blood pressure and is a moderate sedative and hypnotic.

9. Gymnema Sylvestre

Scientific name: Gymnema sylvestre
Common names: Cowplant
Family: Apocynaceae
Origin: India's tropical jungles

Use and Benefits: For about 2,000 years, it has been utilized as a natural diabetes treatment there. The whole plant is being used in decoctions for treating malaria, snake bites, digestive issues, constipation, fever, cough, and urinary diseases, as well as to regulate blood sugar and lower cholesterol.

10. Wild Onion

Scientific name: Allium
Common names: wild onion
Family: Amaryllidaceae
Origin: Europe, North America, North Africa, and Asia

Use and Benefits: Plants can be utilized as decorations, food, seasonings, or medicinal. Colds, asthma, coughs, respiratory ailments, bronchitis, and insect repellent have all been treated with them.

11. Evening Primrose

Scientific name: Oenothera biennis
Common names: Sundrops or Suncups
Family: Onagraceae
Origin: native to South and North America

Use and Benefits: Evening primrose is a flowering plant that has long been used as a food and in herbal medicines. The entire plant has been utilized in decoctions to treat cough, asthma, and other illnesses, as well as to relieve pain. Poultices were also used to help with bruises, swelling, and wound healing. The Navajo and Ramah used it to cure swelling, muscle strain, and throat trouble; the Blackfoot used it for sores and swelling; the Hopi used it as eye medication.

12. Tribulus

Scientific name: Tribulus terrestris
Common names: goats head and puncture vine
Family: Zygophyllaceae
Origin: Africa and south Eurasia

Use and Benefits: For generations, this herb has been utilized in traditional medicine. It can be used for infertility, libido, skin diseases, muscle mass, fertility problems, bladder infections, and as a rinse for oral problems since it contains an active ingredient called steroidal saponins.

13. Bloodroot

Scientific name: Sanguinaria canadensis
Common names: bloodwort, Canada puccoon, red puccoon, redroot, coon root, pauson, and tetterwort
Family: Poppies
Origin: North American woods are home to this species

Use and Benefits: A plant with the name of bloodroot. The rhizome (underground stem) is used in the production of medication. Excessive tooth discomfort may be relieved with the use of a bloodroot. Another common application for it is to treat croup and hoarseness (laryngitis), a painful throat (pharyngitis), and impaired flow in the superficial blood vessels. Antibacterial, anti-inflammatory, and plaque-fighting properties may be found in bloodroot.

14. Skullcap

Scientific name: Scutellaria lateriflora
Common names: Virginian skullcap, hoodwort, blue skullcap, and maddog
Family: mint family
Origin: North America is located in North America.

Use and Benefits: It's also been shown to help with stress relief, nervous system support, +and sleeplessness, tension, and restlessness.

15. Chamomile

Scientific name: Matricaria chamomilla
Common names: German chamomile, chamomile, wild chamomile, Hungarian chamomile, blue chamomile
Family: Asteraceae
Origin: Egypt

Use and Benefits: It's well recognized for being able to be converted into a tea that's widely used to aid sleep. They've also been used to treat gynecological issues, including PMS and cramps, as well as stomach and intestinal cramps, nausea, and stomach flu. It's also a great soothing agent for kids and newborns.

16. Eastern Skunk Cabbage

Scientific name: Symplocarpus Foetidus
Common names: Foetid Pothos, Clumpfoot Cabbage, Meadow Cabbage
Family: Araceae
Origin: native to the eastern United States

Use and Benefits: The Dakota and Winnebago tribes utilized it widely as a medicinal herb to aid in the elimination of mucus in asthma patients. It was used as the medicine "dracontium" in pharmaceutical products from 1820 until 1882 to treat respiratory ailments, neurological disorders, rheumatism, and dropsy.

17. Rabbit Tobacco

Scientific name: Gnaphalium obtusifolium
Common names: Cherokee tobacco, cudweed, Indian posey, sweet everlasting, poverty weed, old field balsam, fussy gussy
Family: Asteraceae
Origin: North America's east coast

Use and Benefits: Native Americans have long utilized it for a range of therapeutic purposes, including colds, cough, asthma, pneumonia, flu, bronchitis, diarrhea, insect repellant, sleep aid, and a variety of other things. It is reported to relieve migraines, sinus difficulties, stomach problems, be a moderate nerve sedative, and improve appetite when used in teas.

18. Honeysuckle

Scientific name: Lonicera
Common names: Japanese honeysuckle
Family: Caprifoliaceae
Origin: North America and Eurasia's northern latitudes

Use and Benefits: Bee stings, asthma, mumps, hepatitis, rheumatoid arthritis, or respiratory infections, such as tumors, pneumonia, skin infections, dysentery, colds, sores, viruses, sore throat, headache, fever, and blood pressure have all been treated with the plant's fruit, juice, stems, flowers, and leaves. Antibacterial, anti-toxin, anti-spasmodic, anti-inflammatory, and purifying activities have also been discovered.

19. Psyllium Seed Husk

Scientific name: Plantago ovata
Common names: Isabgol, Ispaghula, or Psyllium
Family: Plantaginaceae
Origin: India's native

Use and Benefits: Constipation, colon and bowel difficulties, diarrhea, and hemorrhoids have all been documented to be relieved by this fiber-rich supplement. It also aids digestion and is known to help decrease blood cholesterol levels.

20. Indian Hemp

Scientific name: Apocynum Cannabinum
Common names: Amy root, hemp dogbane, American hemp, dogbane, rheumatism root
Family: Apocynaceae
Origin: North America

Use and Benefits: Syphilis, fever, intestinal worms, asthma, rheumatism, and dysentery were all treated using teas made from the plant's cooked roots. It was also used by the Prairie Potawatomi for heart medication and dropsy.

21. Echinacea

Scientific name: Echinacea purpurea
Common names: passionflower, purple coneflower, and coneflower
Family: (Asteraceae) Daisy family
Origin: Eastern North America

Use and Benefits: Plains Indians utilized it to heal illness and wounds, as well as for its general therapeutic properties. Scarlet fever, malaria, syphilis, blood poisoning, tension, earache, insomnia, diphtheria, cough, toothaches, and insect and snake bites are all treated with echinacea. The plant is now used to treat and decrease the duration of common colds and flu, as well as a sore throat and fever. Many herbalists prescribe it to help strengthen immunity and fight infections.

22. Native Hemlock

Scientific name: Tsuga
Common names: eastern hemlock or Canadian hemlock
Family: Pine family
Origin: Eastern and central Canada, as well as the United States.

Use and Benefits: The pitch was commonly used as an ointment or poultice to treat colds and prevent sunburn. Hemorrhages were also treated with a decoction of crushed bark. It has also been used to cure the illness, kidney and bladder disorders, diarrhea, as a mouth and throat gargle, and to wash wounds and ulcers externally.

23. Pau d'arco

Scientific name: Tabebuia avellanedae
Common names: lapacho
Family: Bignonias
Origin: South American native

Use and Benefits: Pain, arthritis, prostate gland inflammation, fever, boils and dysentery, ulcers, and other malignancies have all been treated with it in the past. It has now been discovered that it contains active substances that kill bacteria, fungus, viruses, and parasites. It is infected with influenza.

24. Green Hellebore

Scientific name: Helleborus viridis

Common names: Bear's-foot

Family: Ranunculaceae

Origin: Central and Western Europe

Use and Benefits: Medicine is made from the bulb and root. Despite major safety issues, epilepsy, spasms, fever, high blood pressure, fluid retention, and anxiousness have all been treated using American hellebore

25. Fenugreek

Scientific name: Trigonella foenum-graecum

Common names: bird's foot and Greek hay seed

Family: Fabaceae

Origin: The Mediterranean region, India, Ukraine, and China

Use and Benefits: Fenugreek was utilized by the ancient Egyptians to induce delivery. It's also been used as a digestive aid, a mild cathartic for respiratory issues, dyspepsia, appetite loss, and stomach symptoms. Externally, it was utilized topically to cure swelling, wounds, boils, and eczema. It's been utilized as a moderate antiseptic as well. Recent research has also shown that it is useful in reducing cholesterol and lowering glucose levels in diabetics.

26. White Pine

Scientific name: Pinus strobus

Common names: soft pine and deal pine

Family: Pinaceae

Origin: North American native

Use and Benefits: Native Americans have traditionally employed the young shoots, inner bark, twigs, pitch, and leaves in medical cures for colds, cough, flu, fever, heartburn, headache, osteoarthritis, neuritis, bronchitis, laryngitis, and kidney disorders.

27. Skunk Cabbage

Scientific name: Symplocarpus foetidus
Common names: eastern skunk cabbage or skunk cabbage
Family: Araceae
Origin: North America's east coast

Use and Benefits: Skunk cabbage is being used to cure worms, fungus, and scabies diseases. Cancer, fluid retention, hemorrhage, anxiety, snakebite, skin rashes, splinters, swellings, and injuries are among the other uses

28. Juniper

Scientific name: Juniperus Communis
Common names: Common juniper
Family: Cupressaceae
Origin: Southwest Asia, Europe, and North America

Use and Benefits: Female plants have cones that yield small spherical bluish-black berries that, when completely ripe, were consumed raw or used in teas to heal digestive problems, kidney problems, and bladder problems. It is administered externally as a diluted oil that has a moderate warming effect and has been proven to be beneficial in the treatment of aching joints and wounds.

29. Geranium

Scientific name: Pelargonium
Common names: stork's bill and scented geranium
Family: Geraniaceae
Origin: Eastern Mediterranean region

Use and Benefits: Geranium leaves were being used in teas to cure ulcers and headaches in ancient folk medicine. The Cherokee were known to use a mixture of boiled geranium root and wild grape to wash the mouths of children with thrush in Native American medicine. To treat diarrhea, the Ottawa and Chippewa tribes cooked the whole geranium plant and consumed the tea.

30. Sage

Scientific name: Salvia officinalis
Common names: common sage and garden sage
Family: Lamiaceae
Origin: indigenous to the Mediterranean

Use and Benefits: Because of its powerful purifying properties, sage has long been revered by many Native Americans. Burning sage is supposed to increase overall wellbeing, give equilibrium, cleanse the mind and body of evil spirits, and connect people with the spiritual realm. It has long been used in smudging ceremonies and is claimed to increase intuition, mood, and intellect, as well as fend against negativity and toxins

31. Black Gum

Scientific name: Nyssa sylvatica
Common names: black tupelo, tupelo, sour or black gum
Family: Cornaceae -Dogwood Family
Origin: Eastern North American native

Use and Benefits: This tree's bark has anti-emetic, anti-ophthalmic, and vermifuge properties, all of which may be found in Nyssa sylvatica. Children with worms have received an infusion as a treatment and as a bath additive. When a patient is unable to eat, a powerful decoction is administered to induce vomiting.

32. Saw Palmetto

Scientific name: Serenoas serrulata
Common names: palms
Family: Arecaceae
Origin: North America

Use and Benefits: The palms' heartwood has been ground into flour and utilized for traditional medicinal purposes. Prostate health, It's been used in the treatment of diarrhea, stomach pain, cough, pulmonary congestion, inflammation, sexual vigor, and hunger stimulation.

33. Antelope Sage

Scientific name: Eriogonum jamesii
Common names: James' buckwheat
Family: Polygonaceae
Origin: Southwestern United States native species.

Use and Benefits: For certain of the indigenous peoples of North America, this plant served as a method of birth control. During menstruation, the ladies would take 1 cup of an infusion of the root. Pain during labor has been alleviated by drinking a decoction made from the whole plant. Chewing the root is used to alleviate heart disease and stomach pains. The roots of this plant have been utilized to treat depression using an infusion. The infusion may also be used as an eye wash. Sweetening the saliva has been achieved by chewing on the plant.

34. Sweetgrass

Scientific name: Hierochloe odorata
Common names: Mary's grass, manna grass, or vanilla grass
Family: Poaceae
Origin: north Eurasia and North America

Use and Benefits: Tea made from it has been used to cure a common cold, fever, flu, congestion, sores, and veneral infections. It has been used to treat uterine hemorrhage, placental expulsion after delivery, and miscarriage. Eye infections, blood weakening, edoema, swelling, and chafing were all treated with infusions.

35. Galangal

Scientific name: Alpinia galanga
Common names: Gao liang, blue ginger, and Laos
Family: Zingiberaceae
Origin: Indonesia

Use and Benefits: Like other ginger-related herbs, its use in herbal therapy has long been recognized for its warm and calming effects on digestion. Because of its moderate spicy flavor, it has long been used to alleviate vomiting, abdominal pain, hiccups, diarrhea, flatulence, sore gums, canker sores, and motion sickness.

36. Sumac

Scientific name: Rhus glabra
Common names: scarlet sumac, mountain sumac, smooth sumac, dwarf sumac, upland sumac, vinegar-tree, white shoemake, and red sumac
Family: Anacardiaceae
Origin: North America

Use and Benefits: A decoction of the root or bark was used as an astringent, antiseptic, diuretic, and to treat colds, diarrhea, and fever, as well as to enhance the production of breast milk, treating sore throats, bladder irritation, and uncomfortable urination. An infusion of the plant's root or bark was used as an antibacterial, renal, and for the therapy of colds, diarrhea, fever, increasing breast milk flow, sore lips and throats, bladder irritation, and uncomfortable urination.

37. Yarrow

Scientific name: Achillea millefolium
Common names: old man's pepper, thousand-leaf, nosebleed plant, and devil's nettle
Family: Asteraceae
Origin: Northern Hemisphere

Use and Benefits: Because of its astringent properties, yarrow has been used as a medication for centuries. Inflammation, hemorrhoids, headaches, colds, flu, stomach aches, digestive and urinary systems have all been treated with decoctions. The leaves promote clotting; therefore, it's been recommended for nosebleeds and open wounds or cuts for a long time.

38. Aspen

Scientific name: Populous tremolites
Common names: alamo templon, populous tremella, European aspen, American aspen, trembling aspen, quaking aspen, pulpier faux-tremble, interpupil, popular folium, popular cortex, populous tremolites
Family: Salicaceae (Willow family)
Origin: Native to Central America and Canada (Mexico)

Use and Benefits: High plains, high mountains, and high elevations are the best places to find Aspen because of its tolerance for cold summers and harsh winters. Medicinal uses for the bark and leaves of aspen include alleviating joint, nerve, and urinary tract issues. Aspirin-like compounds, known as silicon, are present, and this has long been recognized as a potent anti-inflammatory agent.

39. White Oak

Scientific name: Quercus alba
Common names: white oak
Family: Fagaceae
Origin: Central and eastern North America

Use and Benefits: Medicine is made from the bark. Tea made from white oak bark is being used to treat arthritis, diarrhea, colds, cough, and bronchitis, as well as to stimulate appetite and improve digestion.

40. Broom Snakeweed

Scientific name: Gutierrezia sarothrae
Common names: broomweed, broom snakeweed, matchweed, and snakeweed
Family: Asteraceae
Origin: Much of western North America, from northern Mexico to western Canada, is home to this species.

Use and Benefits: Numerous characteristics and components of Broom Snakeweed make it an ideal plant for medicinal use. It has antibacterial, antidiuretic, antiasthmatic, and anthelmintic properties, as well as antifungal and antiviral properties. To cure dengue fever, to boost the respiratory system, to assist nursing mothers, and to alleviate stress, it is used in the form of a herbal supplement.

41. Western Hemlock

Scientific name: Tsuga heterophylla
Common names: western hemlock-spruce or western hemlock
Family: Pinaceae
Origin: Native to North America's west coast

Use and Benefits: The bark is diuretic, diaphoretic, and astringent. Hemorrhages, TB, and syphilis have all been treated with a tea of crushed bark. The boiling bark has been used to cure hemorrhages when mixed with licorice fern (Polypodium glycyrrhiza).

42. Garcinia Cambogia

Scientific name: Garcinia Gummi-Gutta
Common names: mangosteen oil tree, gamboge, citrin, tamarind, brindall berry, Malabar
Family: Clusiaceae
Origin: native to Indonesia

Use and Benefits: Swelling, constipation, delayed menstruation, worms, rheumatism, intestinal problems, endurance, energy, gastric ulcers, dysentery, diarrhea, and as a depressant have all been treated with it over the years. Diabetes patients, those with dementia, and pregnant and nursing women are not advised to take this supplement.

43. Passion Flower

Scientific name: Passiflora
Common names: Maypop and Passion Vine
Family: Passifloraceae
Origin: native to the United States

Use and Benefits: anxiety, Insomnia, seizures, hysteria, and epilepsy were all treated using tea made from the leaves and roots. It's also been used in poultices for wounds, boils, and earache, as well as to treat hyperactivity, depression, stress, and muscle soreness. If you're pregnant or breastfeeding, don't take passionflower.

44. Allspice

Scientific name: Pimenta dioica
Common names: Pimento or Jamaica pepper pimenta
Family: Myrtaceae
Origin: the Caribbean and Central American native

Use and Benefits: This spice, as the term says, is a great way to boost your business success and alleviate your mental stress. It boosts willpower and vigor. Money and good fortune spells are other popular uses for it. As a medicinal herb, it may also be used to make a therapeutic herbal bath.

45. Horehound

Scientific name: Marrubium Vulgare
Common names: hog bean, bull's blood, houndsbane, eye of the star, devil's eye, poison tobacco
Family: Lamiaceae
Origin: European native

Use and Benefits: Horehound is used in cough drops and syrups because of its medical usefulness as a cough reliever and expectorant. Constipation, gastrointestinal issues, indigestion, flatulence, and uncomfortable menstruation are among the other applications

46. Uva Ursi

Scientific name: Arctostaphylos uva ursi
Common names: beargrape and bearberry
Family: Ericaceae
Origin: Western North American

Use and Benefits: It was used as a medicine since the 2nd century, and Indigenous People have been known to utilize it to treat urinary and bladder infections. It's also used to treat renal difficulties, menstruation irregularities, cystitis, bloating, diarrhea, hemorrhoids, spleen, and small intestinal abnormalities, as well as to eliminate toxins. Cuts, herpes breakouts, cold sores, and yeast infections have all been treated with it externally.

47. Mullein

Scientific name: Verbascum
Common names: velvet plants
Family: Scrophulariaceae
Origin: Asia and Europe

Use and Benefits: It has a lengthy history of usage as asthma and respiratory illness treatment. Smoke from smoldering mullein leaves and roots was commonly inhaled by Native Americans to relieve chest congestion, asthma attacks, and other respiratory problems.

48. Partridgeberry

Scientific name: Mitchella repens
Common names: deerberry, squaw vine, one-berry, and winter clover
Family: Rubiaceae
Origin: southwest Newfoundland and Minnesota, as well as Florida and Texas.

Use and Benefits: Many Native Americans, especially the Cherokee, brewed tea from the cooked leaves to help with labor in the last weeks of pregnancy. It's also been used to relieve menstrual cramps, control menstruation, and induce delivery.

49. Wild Yam

Scientific name: Dioscorea villosa
Common names: China root, devil's bones, colic root, and Mexican wild yam
Family: Dioscoreaceae
Origin: Eastern North American native

Use and Benefits: Menstrual cramps, poor libido, muscle cramps, colic, menopausal symptoms, dermatitis, rheumatic disorders, and gallbladder problems have all been treated with it in the past.

50. Cattail

Scientific name: Typha latifolia
Common names: reedmace, bullrush, corndog grass, & punks
Family: Typhaceae
Origin: South and North America, Eurasia, Europe, and Africa are among the places where this species may be found.

Use and Benefits: Poultices for burns, sprains, wound infection, edema, and boils were employed in Indigenous American herbal therapy. Abdominal pains, whooping cough, kidney stones, gonorrhea, cysts, and diarrhea were all treated with it internally.

BOOK 18

HERBAL MEDICINES & PLANT REMEDIES. - VOLUME 2

1. Bee Pollen

Scientific name: Bee Pollen
Common names: bee bread and ambrosia

Use and Benefits: Bee pollen is the floral pollen that gathers on the bodies and legs of worker bees. Bee saliva and nectar may also be used in the mix. Bee pollen is widely used as a food source. It is also utilized orally to increase hunger, stamina, and physical performance, as well as to slow down the aging process. Ingestion of bee pollen may assist boost the immune system, while the topical application may aid in wound healing. The exact mechanism through which bee pollen has these benefits is still a mystery. Some individuals believe that bee pollen's enzymes may be used as medication. Similar enzymes, on the other hand, are digested in the stomach; therefore, it is doubtful that consuming pollen enzymes through the mouth produces these effects.

2. Ragleaf Bahia

Scientific name: Bahia Dissecta
Common names: yellow ragleaf or yellow ragweed
Family: Daisy family
Origin: The southwest United States

Use and Benefits: Yellow ragleaf is used for the treatment of the heart and kidneys. Root tea is used as a contraceptive.

3. Horse Gentian

Scientific name: Triosteum aurantiacum
Common names: Orange-fruited horse
Family: Caprifoliaceae
Origin: Eastern Asia and North America

Use and Benefits: Horse gentians have long been prized for their therapeutic qualities. Native Americans used them to treat bladder pain and applied them topically to wounds and inflamed areas. Fevers were treated with roots, which also served as a potent laxative. When dried, the berries can be utilized as a coffee substitute.

4. Plantain

Scientific name: Plantago major

Common names: white man's foot, ripple grass, snakeweed, waybread, cuckoo's bread, Englishman's foot

Family: Plantaginaceae

Origin: Northern and Central Asia, as well as Europe, are home to this species.

Use and Benefits: The seeds and leaves were used as a poultice to heal battle wounds, ulcers, insect bites, bronchitis, T.B, sore throat, urinary infections, laryngitis, digestive issues, and as a blood-purifying tonic. The herb's root was used to treat toothaches, and the juice was used to treat earaches.

5. Wild Black Cherry

Scientific name: Prunus serotina

Common names: mountain black cherry, rum cherry, black choke, and black cherry

Family: Rosaceae

Origin: Eastern North American native

Use and Benefits: Cough, "blood tonic," fevers, common cold, flu, laryngitis, whooping cough, bronchitis, breathing problems, hypertension, colic, edoema, arthritis, diarrhea, lung ailments, eye swelling, swollen lymph nodes, tuberculosis, inflammation-related fever diseases, and dyspepsia were all treated with the dried inner bark in tea or syrup.

6. Buffaloberry

Scientific name: Shepherdia

Common names: blueberry, soapberry, chaparral berry, rabbitberry, soopolallie, and silver leaf

Family: Elaeagnaceae

Origin: This species is found throughout the north and west of North America.

Use and Benefits: Plant and berry parts were used to cure constipation, TB and a host of other ailments, including gynecological and gynecological issues as well as a host of other ailments including gynecological and gynecological issues. Buffaloberries are edible, but they have a strong sour flavor and might leave your mouth feeling dry after eating them.

7. Astragalus

Scientific name: Astragalus propinquus
Common names: locoweed, milkvetch (most species), and goat's-thorn
Family: Fabaceae
Origin: Originally from the eastern part of Asia

Use and Benefits: Astragalus, often known as "the young person's ginseng," boosts the immune response and aids in the regeneration of the bone marrow book, which serves as the body's natural defense. It's an excellent plant for addressing longterm imbalances. It's also useful for those with diabetes since it regulates the breakdown of dietary carbohydrates.

8. Persimmon

Scientific name: Diospyros
Common names: persimmon
Family: Ebenaceae
Origin: China

Use and Benefits: They've also been used in teas for a long time in traditional Asian medicine to treat hiccups, bedwetting, constipation, fever, and enhance circulation. They've also been shown to help prevent heart attacks, strokes, and hypertension by reducing fluid retention.

9. Dandelion

Scientific name: Taraxacum officinale
Common names: common weed
Family: Asteraceae
Origin: North American native

Use and Benefits: Its leaves, roots, and flowers are all high in multiple vitamins and also minerals like potassium, iron, and zinc. Its roots are used in coffee replacements, while the flowers are used to manufacture specific wines. Dandelion leaves and roots were used in traditional medicine to treat liver disorders, renal illness, edema, skin problems, stomach discomfort, and heartburn.

10. Thistle

Scientific name: Silybum adans

Common names: Mediterranean thistle, milk thistle, Marian thistle, Mary thistle, and holy thistle

Family: Daisy family

Origin: Native to North Africa, Europe, and the Middle East's Mediterranean regions

Use and Benefits: It has been used to treat chronic hepatic disease and protects the liver from poisons for over 2,000 years. Hepatitis, cancer, and excessive cholesterol have all been controlled with it.

11. Ashwagandha

Scientific name: Withania somnifera

Common names: poison gooseberry, Indian ginseng, or Winter cherry

Family: Solanaceae

Origin: Native to the continent of North America (Montana, Alaska, Oregon, Nevada, Utah)

Use and Benefits: Aromatically, Ashwagandha's root is said to be tonic and analgesic; it is also narcotic and diuretic; it is anthelmintic; it is thermogenic, and it is stimulating. Emaciation of youngsters, old age, rheumatoid arthritis, vitiated states of leukoderma, vata, constipation, sleeplessness and neurological breakdown are some of the ailments in which it is widely used to treat. In order to alleviate joint inflammation, a paste made from water and crushed roots is applied topically.

12. Rose Hip

Scientific name: Rosa canina

Common names: rose haw

Family: Rosaceae

Origin: the Middle East and Europe

Use and Benefits: Rosehips have been used in meals and herbal medicines for a long time. Teas have been used to cure depressions, spasms, and inflammation, as well as to relieve a cough, urinary tract difficulties, renal disorders, diarrhea, and as an astringent.

13. Arnica

Scientific name: Arnica montana
Common names: mountain arnica, wolf's bane, leopard's bane, and mountain tobacco
Family: Asteraceae
Origin: Native to the continent of North America (Montana, Alaska, Oregon, Nevada, Utah)

Use and Benefits: Arnica is an effective painkiller, but unlike other medicines, it does not lead to addiction. Muscle-related ailments may also be treated using the leaves. It reduces inflammation and alleviates pain and swelling in the joints. Using homeopathic arnica solutions is the most effective method. Before consuming it, let it disperse over time.

14. White Willow

Scientific name: Salix alba
Common names: white willow
Family: Salicaceae
Origin: Europe, as well as western and central Asia, is home to this species.

Use and Benefits: Willow bark has been used for thousands of years, dating back to Hippocrates' (400 BC) advice to patients chewing on the bark to relieve fever and inflammation. It's been used for a long time to treat pain, including low back pain, headaches, and inflammatory disorders, including bursitis and tendinitis.

15. Rooibos

Scientific name: Aspalathus linearis
Common names: Red Bush
Family: Crassulaceae
Origin: South African native

Use and Benefits: Teas containing it have long been used to treat psychological tension, allergies, digestive issues, newborn colic, asthma, heartburn, nausea, and skin diseases.

16. Valerian Root

Scientific name: Valeriana officinalis

Common names: all-heal and garden heliotrope,

Family: Caprifoliaceae

Origin: Europe and West Asia

Use and Benefits: It's been used for sedation, intestinal colic, hysteria stress, cramps, restlessness, gastrointestinal pain, anxiety, and irritable bowel syndrome for centuries.

17. Buckwheat

Scientific name: Fagopyrum esculentum

Common names: common buckwheat

Family: Polygonaceae

Origin: Its origins are supposed to be in China.

Use and Benefits: Historically, it's been consumed as a meal and utilized as an herbal remedy. Blood pressure is lowered, the arteries are strengthened, and it is used to treat diarrhea, dysentery and skin sores, as well as many circulation issues.

18. Stoneseed

Scientific name: Lithospermum officinale

Common names: gromwell

Family: Boraginaceae

Origin: west Canada and the western United States

Use and Benefits: The mature seeds were long being crushed into a fine powder and were utilized to cure bladder stones and arthritis. Its roots were also utilized as a contraceptive by several Native Americans, including the Shoshoni. Eruptive disorders like measles, smallpox, and itch were treated with a syrup produced from an infusion of the stems and roots.

19. Blackberry

Scientific name: Rubus fruticosus

Common names: blackberry, bramble, black heg, European blackberry, wild blackberry

Family: Rosaceae

Origin: Predominantly found in the northern hemisphere

Use and Benefits: For more than 2,000 years, Europeans have relied on blackberries for medicinal reasons. As a remedy for oral diseases, bleeding gums, and cancerous lesions, they would eat the leaves or make tea from blackberry shoots. In animals, polyphenol antioxidants, which are naturally occurring compounds, have been shown to boost key metabolic processes. The blackberry root, which is also an astringent, is also used in herbal therapy to treat diarrhea and dysentery.

20. Jiaogulan

Scientific name: Gynostemma pentaphyllum
Common names: Southern Ginseng and Twisting-vine Orchid
Family: Cucurbitaceae
Origin: Asia

Use and Benefits: It has numerous health-promoting and anti-aging properties. It has been discovered to high blood pressure and lower cholesterol, enhance immune systems, limit cancer growth, enhance digestive and reproductive systems, mental and hepatic functioning, and stress-related symptoms, among other things.

21. Eleuthero

Scientific name: Eleutherococcus senticosus
Common names: wild pepper, devil's bush, Siberian ginseng, devil's shrub, prickly Eleutherococcus, pepperbush, touch-me-not
Family: Araliaceae
Origin: native to Northeast Asia, Korean Peninsula, and southeastern Siberia.

Use and Benefits: Its dried roots have long been used to cure colds, flu, weariness, and edoema, as well as to improve concentration and focus, strengthen the immune system, and boost stamina. Before utilizing, people who are taking medication for increased blood pressure should check their doctor. Take it a few hours before night to avoid insomnia.

22. Oak

Scientific name: Quercus robur
Common names: common oak
Family: Fagaceae

Origin: Northern Hemisphere.

Use and Benefits: Acorns are an excellent diet for people suffering from degenerative, wasting diseases like tuberculosis, and acorn porridge was frequently given when the disease was widespread in the early 1800s. The (inner) bark of the oak was used to prepare a bitter decoction that was used to sore throats, cure diarrhea, kidney and bladder disorders, infections, and monthly bleeding among Native Americans. Skin issues, ringworm, burns, wounds, sprains, and edoema were all treated using poultices.

23. Wheat Grass

Scientific name: Triticum aestivum
Common names: wheatgrass
Family: Poaceae
Origin: all around the North Temperate Zone

Use and Benefits: Wheatgrass has been shown to increase energy levels, enhance the immune system, and inhibit the progression of many cancers. Bronchitis, cough, the common cold, infection, anemia, and fever have all been treated with it.

24. Atractylodes

Scientific name: Atractylodes
Common names: Atractylis ovata, Atractylis lancea, and Atractylode blanc
Family: Asteraceae
Origin: Eastern Asian in origin

Use and Benefits: Administering Atractylodes may help with nausea and vomiting caused by cancer treatment as well as other conditions such as intolerance to dust mites and joint discomfort (rheumatism). When the kidneys fail, a mechanical way of "cleaning the blood" known as dialysis is used to treat lung cancer and dialysis-related problems.

25. Willow

Scientific name: Salix
Common names: osiers and sallows

Family: Salicaceae

Origin: The Northern Hemisphere's temperate zones

Use and Benefits: It was a common medical therapy for Native Americans all over the American continent. This is due to the presence of Salicin, a chemically similar component to aspirin found in willows. Pain, headaches, toothaches, mouth sores, stomach disorders, and diarrhea have all been treated with it.

26. Sweet Everlasting

Scientific name: Pseudognaphalium obtusifolium

Common names: rabbit tobacco, old field balsam, and sweet everlasting

Family: Asteraceae

Origin: North America's east coast

Use and Benefits: Sedative, astringent, diuretic, cold-symptom and pain reducer are some of the medicinal uses. This plant seems like a therapeutic marvel, and when crushed, it even smells like maple syrup!

27. Buckthorn

Scientific name: Rhamnus

Common names: buckthorns

Family: Rhamnaceae

Origin: mostly found in eastern Asia and northern America

Use and Benefits: Buckthorn bark is the only part of the plant used medicinally. When used as a purgative or laxative, Buckthorn has been used medicinally since the 14th century. While it's most often known for its role in the treatment of skin conditions, including eczema and seborrheic dermatitis, it's also been used to treat liver health issues like obesity.

28. Blue Cohosh

Scientific name: Caulophyllum thalictroides

Common names: squaw-root, blue cohosh, Caulophyllum fauxpigamon, papoose-root

Family: Berberidaceae

Origin: Eastern North American native (Oklahoma east, Manitoba, Atlantic Ocean).

Use and Benefits: A plant is known as blue cohosh. Algonquin Indians used the term "rough" to describe the look of the roots of cohosh. Medicine is made from the root. Blue cohosh is a dangerous plant. However, the supplement is still accessible. The supplements may not have any warnings at all. Blue cohosh may have estrogen-like actions, according to some researchers. As a result, it may cause a reduction in blood flow to the heart, which may lead to a decrease in blood oxygenation in the heart.

29. Wild Ginger

Scientific name: Asarum canadense
Common names: Canadian snakeroot and Canada wild ginger
Family: Aristolochiaceae
Origin: Eastern North American woodlands are home to this species.

Use and Benefits: The roots were used to treat diarrhea, digestive issues, enlarged breasts, cough, and colds, scarlet fever, nerves, cramps, earache, headache, convulsions, tuberculosis, urinary problems, and venereal illness by Native Americans. It was also utilized as a stimulant and hunger booster.

30. Spirulina

Scientific name: Arthrospira platensis
Common names: blue-green algae
Family: Microcoleaceae
Origin: Mexico's center region
Use and Benefits: A form of blue-green algae high in protein, minerals, vitamins, and antioxidants that helps to enhance immunity and prevent allergic reactions. It's also supposed to help with infections, liver problems, and some types of cancer.

31. Peppermint

Scientific name: Mentha piperita
Common names: Peppermint
Family: Lamiaceae
Origin: the Middle East and Europe

Use and Benefits: It has a lengthy history of therapeutic use, dating back at least ten thousand years, according to archaeological data. It has traditionally been used to ease an upset stomach, heartburn and help indigestion. It is most commonly used as a flavor for gum toothpaste and tea. It has been used to cure skin irritations, headaches, depression, anxiety, nausea, diarrhea, menstrual cramps, and bloating because of its relaxing and numbing impact. It's been used to treat colds externally in the form of chest rubs.

32. Senna Leaves

Scientific name: Satureja
Common names: summer savory, mountain savory and winter savory
Family: Fabaceae
Origin: all over the tropics

Use and Benefits: Spleen, liver, anemia, cholera, typhoid, jaundice, gout, rheumatism, tumors, bronchitis, leprosy, skin problems, dyspepsia, and cough are all conditions that it can aid with.

33. Catnip/Catmint

Scientific name: Nepeta cataria
Common names: catswort, catnip, catmint, & catwort
Family: Lamiaceae
Origin: Asia, Europe, and Africa are home to this species.

Use and Benefits: The plant has a rich history of therapeutic usage for its calming qualities, as well as a mild numbing effect. Teas, poultices, and smoking are all ways to utilize it. Fresh or dried stems and leaves are used to prepare a fragrant herb tea that has been shown to help with digestive problems, fever reduction, cold and flu treatment, and newborn colic. It's also been shown to help with anxiety and restlessness.

34. Kava Kava

Scientific name: Piperm methysticum
Common names: Kew, Kawa, Yagona, and Sakau
Family: Piperaceae
Origin: Islands of the Pacific

Use and Benefits: The plant's roots are most typically used to make a sedative or anesthetic drink. Some people eat the root to get relief from throat aches. Anxiety and sleeplessness are also treated with this herb.

35. Wild Lettuce

Scientific name: Lactuca virosa
Common names: opium lettuce, green endive, and acrid lettuce
Family: Asteraceae
Origin: Native to North America.

Use and Benefits: Dropsy, colic, sleeplessness, cough, stress, and anxiety have all been treated with it.

36. Cedar

Scientific name: Cedrus
Common names: cedar
Family: Pinaceae
Origin: The Mediterranean area and the western Himalayas are home to this species.

Use and Benefits: It was used in teas to treat respiratory problems, joint discomfort, flatulence, water retention, enhance hunger and digestion, coughs, fungal infections, fevers, colds, and flu. Wounds, hair loss, skin rashes, acne, eczema, fungal infections, warts, aching joints, hemorrhoids, leprosy, syphilis, and on the chest for asthma were all treated with it in salves and oils. Tuberculosis is treated with cedar leaves, while chest infections, sleeplessness, and diabetes are treated with a cedar decoction.

37. Milk-vetch

Scientific name: Astragalus
Common names: locoweed, milkvetch and goat's-thorn
Family: Fabaceae
Origin: native to the Northern Hemisphere's temperate zones

Use and Benefits: Milkvetch root has been used as a medication in China for over 2000 years and has been shown to improve immunological function, protect the liver, stimulate urine, fight age and stress, lower blood pressure, and resist bacteria.

38. Cascara Sagrada

Scientific name: Rhamnus purshiana
Common names: bearberry, California buckthorn, & yellow bark
Family: Rhamnaceae
Origin: From southern Canada to central California & inland to western

Use and Benefits: Montana, this tree is endemic to western North America. It is primarily prescribed for the treatment of gastrointestinal disorders. A powerful laxative, it is also thought to strengthen the walls of the colon. Tea can be brewed from the dried bark, but it has a bitter flavor. Because fresh cascara bark can cause vomiting and bloody diarrhea, it should not be consumed. Aged at least a year or subjected to a particular heat treatment is required.

39. Boneset

Scientific name: Eupatorium perfoliatum
Common names: ague weed, Indian sage, Agueweed, thoroughwort, Crosswort, Eupatoire, or Bois Perfolié
Family: Asteraceae
Origin: native to the United States and Canada's east coasts

Use and Benefits: Boneset is a kind of plant that grows in the Mediterranean region. There are several medicinal uses for dried leaves and blossoms. Analgesia, vomiting, and constipation may all be treated with boneset. It is also used as a stimulant and to induce sweating in the treatment of bronchitis, swine flu, bronchitis, inflammation of the nasal passages (rheumatism), joint discomfort (rheumatism), dengue fever, fluid retention, and pneumonia.

40. Fendler's Bladderpod

Scientific name: Lesquerella fendleri
Common names: yellowtop, Lesquerella praecox, Lesquerella foliacea
Family: Brassicaceae (Mustard Family)

Origin: Indigenous to the Southwest US and northern Mexico.

Use and Benefits: Native Americans, particularly the Hopi, employed the root for a range of purposes, including snakebite treatment, gynecological help after childbirth, and vomiting induction. A poultice made from the roots was administered to painful eyes by the Kayenta and Navajo tribes. It was also used as a nasal snuff, a toothache poultice, and to cure spider bites.

41. Chokecherry

Scientific name: Prunus virginiana
Common names: Black Chokecherry, Western Chokecherry, and Wild Cherry
Family:
Origin: native to the US and Canada

Use and Benefits: It was regarded as one of the most significant native medications, alongside Sassafras, in early American medicine. Smallpox, the discomfort of the chest and neck, scurvy, cough, lung hemorrhages, bowel inflammation, colds, stomach cramps, diarrhea, digestive issues, cholera, sores, gangrenous wounds, aches, wounds, and severe burns were all treated with the tree's bark.

42. Lavender

Scientific name: Lavandula
Common names: English lavender
Family: Lamiaceae
Origin: the Canary Islands and Cape Verde

Use and Benefits: The lavender essential oil has antibacterial and anti-inflammatory effects; hair loss, Insomnia, anxiety, melancholy, headache, exhaustion, stress, and surgical pain have all been linked to it. It was used to sterilize floors and walls in hospitals during World War I. Infusions were used to treat burns, insect bites, and acne on the skin.

43. Pinon

Scientific name: Penus edulis
Common names: pinyon
Family: Pine family

Origin: native to the United States

Use and Benefits: Inhaling smoke from needles or burning resin was used to treat cough for medicinal purposes. The Navajo people used a salve made of buds to treat burns and used hot resin to eradicate facial hair.

44. Rosemary

Scientific name: Rosmarinus officinalis
Common names: rosemary and Romero
Family: Mint family
Origin: indigenous to the Mediterranean

Use and Benefits: It has traditionally been used to boost memory, reduce muscle discomfort and spasms, promote hair growth, and strengthen the circulatory and neural systems, as well as for culinary uses. It is also thought to strengthen the immune system, increase menstrual flow, serve as an abortifacient, alleviate dyspepsia, and increase menstrual flow. It may also have anti-cancer qualities, as well as benefits for the liver and the treatment of infections.

45. Cayenne

Scientific name: Capsicum
Common names: hot pepper, chili pepper, tabasco pepper, red pepper, Mexican chili, pimiento
Family: nightshade family -Solanaceae
Origin: the Americas' indigenous species

Use and Benefits: It's used as a meal as well as a medicine, and it's well recognized for treating circulatory and intestinal disorders. Rheumatism, arthritis, diabetes, shingles, heart disease, stomach issues, chronic nerve pain, headaches, varicose veins, menstrual cramps, and asthma were among the other illnesses for which it was prescribed. It was also used to treat throat irritation with a gargle. It was used to dull the pain and improve blood flow in wounds. It's been used to treat cholesterol and high blood pressure in recent years.

46. Chlorella

Scientific name: Chlorella pyrenoidosa
Common names: green algae

Family: Chlorellaceae

Origin: indigenous to the United States

Use and Benefits: A genus of single-celled green algae with anti-tumor capabilities and efficacy in preventing cancer, immune response support, weight management, high blood pressure reduction, cholesterol reduction, and wound healing.

47. Hellebores

Scientific name: Helleborus

Common names: bugbane, witchweed, earth gall, devil's bite, Indian poke, and tickleweed

Family: Ranunculaceae

Origin: Europe and Asia

Use and Benefits: It has been used in traditional medicinal cures for a long time, but it is no longer employed because the herb has been proven to be extremely toxic and to have multiple serious side effects, even at therapeutic doses. Internally, American Hellebore has been used to treat peritonitis, pneumonia, pain, asthma, colds, cholera, epilepsy, croup, consumption, fever, hypertension, dyspepsia, herpes, gout, headache, whooping cough, inflammation, sciatica, rheumatism, shingles, scrofulous, toothache, tumors, and typhus in the past.

48. Star Anise

Scientific name: Illicium verum

Common names: Star Anise

Family: Schisandraceae

Origin: Asia

Use and Benefits: It's been used to treat colic, flatulence, rheumatism, headache, nausea, vomiting, stomach distress, flu, cough, and whooping cough in new moms, as well as to promote appetite, help digestion, and boost milk production. Some folk cures advocate it to aid in childbirth, boost libido, and reduce menopausal symptoms.

49. Lecithin

Use and Benefits: Saturated fatty acids (SFAs) are a type of yellow-brown fatty compounds that can be found in plant and animal tissues. They can be found in foods such as eggs and peanut butter. It has been discovered to be particularly beneficial to the heart and brain systems' health. Supplements are also supposed to help with the nervous and vascular systems, as well as indigestion

50. Black Cohosh

Scientific name: Actaea racemosa
Common names: black cohosh, fairy candle, or black snakeroot
Family: Ranunculaceae
Origin: indigenous to North America

Use and Benefits: Medicinally, the root may be utilized to treat estrogen-related issues. Black cohosh has the potential to boost estrogen's effects in certain people. It's possible that black cohosh might reduce estrogen's effects in other sections of the human body. No, black cohosh isn't a "herbal estrogen" or alternative for estrogen. Premenstrual syndrome, menopause, weak and brittle bones, painful menstruation, and many other ailments are among the conditions for which black cohosh is often used; however, there are no studies to prove any of these claims.

BOOK 19

HERBAL MEDICINES & PLANT REMEDIES. - VOLUME 3

1. TOBACCO

SCIENTIFIC NAME: NICOTIANA

COMMON NAME: TOBACCO

FAMILY: SOLANACEAE

ORIGIN: AUSTRALIA AND AMERICA ARE HOME TO THIS SPECIES.

USE AND BENEFITS:

The leaves of the plant have long been practiced to treat pain, colic, renal difficulties, dropsy, fever, colic, convulsions, fever, toothache, poison, skin disorders, boils, TB, vertigo, and bug and snake bites. It doesn't have to be smoked to have spiritual effects, and it's often used in purifying ceremonies.

2. OLIVE OIL

SCIENTIFIC NAME: OLEA EUROPAEA (OLIVE PLANT)
COMMON NAME: COMMON OLIVE
FAMILY: OLEACEAE
ORIGIN: MEDITERRANEAN BASIN
USE AND BENEFITS:

Olive oil is a liquid fat made from olives that are extracted by pressing whole olives. Olive oil has been utilized in cooking, pharmaceuticals, cosmetics, soaps, and also as a fuel for ancient oil lamps for a long time. It has long been used in cooking and traditional medicine due to its high amount of fats and anti-oxidative compounds. When used in food, olive oil aids digestion and prevents constipation

3. Creosote Bush

Scientific name: Larrea tridentata
Common names: Spanish hediondo & Hediondilla
Family: Zygophyllaceae
Origin: A common sight in the deserts in the south and west of the United States.

Use and Benefits: Respiratory disorders, sexually transmitted illnesses, TB, dysmenorrhea, chickenpox, and snakebite are all treated with it. Sadly, the U.S. Food & Drug Authority has issued health warnings regarding the dangers of swallowing chaparral today, claiming that it may cause kidney and liver damage.

4. Ginseng

Scientific name: Ginseng
Common names: Siberian ginseng, panax ginseng, and American ginseng
Family: Araliaceae
Origin: Korea, China, and Russia

Use and Benefits: For thousands of years, it has been an essential herbal therapy in traditional Chinese medicine, primarily as a remedy for weakness and exhaustion. It has also been utilized for a variety of other conditions over the years, including sexual dysfunction in men, diabetes, stress reduction, increased energy, improved memory, and immune system stimulation. Specific impacts that assist the nervous system, lung function, liver function, and circulatory system have been discovered through research. The root is most commonly accessible in dried form, whether whole or diced; however, Ginseng stems and leaves are also utilized in dried form, though they are not as prized.

5. Palo Santo

Scientific name: Bursera graveolens
Common names: palo santo
Family: Burseraceae
Origin: South and Central America

Use and Benefits: Palo Santo tea has been used to treat arthritis, headaches, sore throats, colds, and flu as well as a natural digestive aid and anti-inflammatory. It is also supposed to help in faster recovery from disease by supporting the nervous and immune systems.

6. Oat Straw

Scientific name: Avena sativa
Common names: Groats, Oatgrass, Herb Oats, and Wild Oats.
Family: Poaceae
Origin: North America and Northern Europe

Use and Benefits: Since prehistoric times, oats have been an essential source of food for both people and animals. It's also been used for a long time to treat a variety of medical issues, including cholesterol reduction, increased vigor and stamina, anxiousness, tiredness, sleeplessness, and digestive issues. It has recently been discovered to be beneficial in the treatment of multiple sclerosis. ADHD, cancer, tumors, and diabetes are just a few examples.

7. Eucalyptus

Scientific name: Eucalyptus Globulus
Common names: southern blue gum, Tasmanian blue gum, or blue gum
Family: Myrtaceae
Origin: Australian

Use and Benefits: Eucalyptus oil produced from the leaves was used for cleaning, deodorising, and in very small amounts in food additives such sweets, cough drops, toothpaste, and decongestants over the years. It also works as an insect repellant. Traditional Aboriginal treatments employed eucalyptus oil-based topical ointments to treat wounds, fungal infections, swelling, arthritis, and skin disorders, while teas have small amounts of dried leaves were used to treat fevers, coughs, colds, bronchitis, sore throats, and sinusitis. The fumes were sometimes used for similar purposes. Its applications quickly extended over the globe. It's still used as an antiseptic to treat diabetes and may be found in a variety of lozenges, syrups, cough, rubs, and vapour baths across the US and Europe.

8. Elderberries

Scientific name: Sambucus nigra

Common names: black elder, elderberry, European elder
Family: Adoxaceae
Origin: Europe and North America

Use and Benefits: Elderberry berries and blooms are high in antioxidants and vitamins, which may help to enhance your immune system. They may be able to reduce inflammation, reduce stress, and protect your heart. Constipation, epilepsy, headaches, kidney difficulties, fever, muscle and joint pain have all been treated with it.

9. Hops

Scientific name: Humulus lupulus
Common names: strobiles or seed cones
Family: Cannabaceae
Origin: Europe and Asia.

Use and Benefits: They were also utilized for a range of ailments in ancient herbal therapy. It's been used for centuries as a tension reliever, digestive aid and sleep aid due to its bitter components. They were also used to cure anxiety, restlessness and ease muscles. They were sometimes taken alone, but most commonly in combination with other herbs.

10. Hawthorn

Scientific name: Crataegus
Common names: hawthorn, thornapple, whitethorn, quickthorn, Maytree,
or hawberry
Family: Rosaceae
Origin: Europe, Asia, Northern Africa, and North America are all temperate areas of the Northern Hemisphere

Use and Benefits: Since the 1st century, hawthorn has been utilized to treat cardiac problems. By the early 1800s, it was being used by American doctors to treat circulatory and respiratory ailments. The berries were traditionally used to treat cardiac disorders such as irregular pulse, chest pain, high blood pressure, artery hardening, and heart failure.

11. Gentiana

Scientific name: Gentiana

Common names: bitter root, gal weed, bitter wort, longdan, yellow gentian, snakeroot, Sampsons and qin jiao

Family: Gentianaceae

Origin: Asia, Europe, and the Americas

Use and Benefits: It was frequently utilized by Indigenous People to heal digestive disorders and as an appetite enhancer, despite its exceedingly bitter taste. Numerous species were also utilized to treat Malaria, promote menstruation, and eliminate worms from the body. It was also applied to wounds and severe inflammation as a topical treatment.

12. Prickly Pear Cactus

Scientific name: OpuntiaeEngelmanni

Common names: cow's tongue cactus, Texas prickly pear and desert prickly pear

Family: Cactaceae

Origin: Northern Mexico and the southwestern United States

Use and Benefits: Native Americans ate the younger pads, while the older ones were utilized as a poultice for injuries, burns, boils, stopping bleeding, and swelling prostates. Teas were used to curing infections, TB, and the immune system internally. It has also been shown to help with cholesterol reduction and the prevention of diet-related heart problems and adult-onset diabetes.

13. Licorice Root

Scientific name: Glycyrrhiza glabra

Common names: sweet root, licorice, and gan zao (Chinese licorice)

Family: Apiaceae

Origin: Asia and Southern Europe

Use and Benefits: It has been used for the treatment of stomach ulcers, bronchitis, heartburn, sore throats, hepatitis, colic, liver diseases, malaria, TB, food poisoning, and chronic fatigue syndrome over the years.

14. Milkweed

Scientific name: Asclepias syriaca
Common names: common silkweed, cottonweed, common milkweed, wild cotton, silkweed
Family: Apocynaceae
Origin: Africa, North and South America

Use and Benefits: Backache was treated with an infusion of milkweed root and Virgin's Bower (Clematis species). The plant was also employed as an antidote for dropsy, laxative, and a root infusion for sexual disorders. Treatment for vaginal troubles, stomach problems, chest discomfort, and topically on ringworm, warts, and bee stings were among the other uses.

15. Raspberry

Scientific name: Rubus idaeus
Common names: red raspberry
Family: Rosaceae
Origin: European native

Use and Benefits: It can be used as an astringent to treat a variety of ailments, including diarrhea and mouth problems such as mouth sores and inflammation. Gargle to relieve sore throats. For stomach symptoms and moderate nausea, fresh and dried leaves were steeped in tea.

16. Fennel

Scientific name: Foeniculum Vulgare
Common names: fennel
Family: Apiaceae
Origin: The Mediterranean coasts

Use and Benefits: Fennel was used as a digestive aid in Puritan folk medicine. The leaves, roots, and seeds of fennel are harmless and edible, but the essential oil collected from the seeds could be hazardous, even in little amounts. It's been used for years for a digestive aid, flatulence cure, appetite stimulant, and to help nursing women produce more breast milk. Teas and tonics made from the leaves and seeds were used to cure stomach pains, newborn colic, coughs, colds, respiratory issues, and constipation.

17. Witch Hazel

Scientific name: Hamamelis virginiana
Common names: witch hazels
Family: Hamamelidaceae
Origin: North America is located in North America.

Use and Benefits: To cure painful muscles, cuts, bug bites, skin irritations, bruises, and to halt bleeding, Witch Hazel extract was prepared by boiling the shrub's stems.

18. St. John's Wort

Scientific name: Hypericum perforatum
Common names: Tipton's weed, Klamath weed or chase-devil
Family: Hypericaceae
Origin: Europe, North Africa, and western Asia

Use and Benefits: The most prevalent usage of St. John's Wort is as an antidepressant. It's also been used to treat muscle pain, as well as sprains, cramps, varicose veins, bruises, menopausal symptoms, and anxiety.

19. Rhodiola

Scientific name: Rhodiola rosea
Common names: Golden Root, Roseroot, Aaron's Rod
Family: Crassulaceae
Origin: Asia, Europe, and North America

Use and Benefits: It's been used for a long time to lift one's spirits and relieve despair. It's also been shown to boost mental and physical performance, as well as reduce fatigue, stress, and anxiety.

20. Marshmallow Leaf/Root

Scientific name: Althea officinalis
Common names: marshmallow plant, white mallow, mallow, common marshmallow
Family: Malvaceae

Origin: Europe and Western Asia

Use and Benefits: Marshmallow coats the skin and the walls of the digestive tract with a protective layer. It also includes compounds that may help heal wounds and reduce cough. External applications have been shown to help with edoema, cuts, boils, wounds, eczema, and psoriasis.

21. Club Moss

Scientific name: Lycopodiopsida
Common names: foxtail, clubfoot moss, running club moss, ground pine, vegetable sulfur, staghorn, and wolf's claw
Family: Lycopodiopsida
Origin: Eurasia and Northern North America are home to chilly woodlands and Alpine Alps.

Use and Benefits: The use of club moss as a medicine date back to the Middle Ages in Europe. Vegetable Sulfur's previous name alludes to the powder's extremely flammable oil. It has been used as a diuretic in the treatment of kidney stones and urinary tract infections.

22. Sarsaparilla

Scientific name: Smilax regelii
Common names: Honduran sarsaparilla, sarsaparilla, and Jamaican sarsaparilla
Family: Smilacaceae
Origin: Central America

Use and Benefits: Syphilis, digestion, pain, blood purification, arthritis, colds, impotence, gonorrhea, rheumatism, wounds, fever, cold, hypertension, skin infections, leprosy, and cancer are just a few of the medical uses for this Central American native. It has anti-oxidant qualities, just like many other plants.

23.Lemongrass

Scientific name: Cymbopogon
Common names: Barbed Wire Grass, Citronella Grass, Silky Heads, and Fever Grass
Family: Poaceae
Origin: Warm tropical and temperate climates

Use and Benefits: It has been widely utilized as a herb in Asian food, including teas, soups, and curries, in addition to its therapeutic benefits. It's also been employed both as a pesticide and preservation due to its antifungal effects. In medicine, just the dried and fresh leaves of lemongrass, as well as the essential oil extracted from them, are used to treat coughs, wounds, asthma, and bladder problems. It helps to reduce headaches and encourages perspiration.

24. Saltbush

Scientific name: Atriplex
Common names: saltbush and orache
Family: Amaranthaceae
Origin: Australia, South and North America, and Eurasia

Use and Benefits: Pain, blisters, insect and spider bites, rashes, stomach problems, and other ailments have all been treated with various species for centuries. It's used to purify the water as well. The Navajo were known to use the leaves for discomfort, cough, gastrointestinal disorders, and toothache relief, in addition to insect bites.

25. Lemon Balm

Scientific name: Melissa officinalis
Common names: lemon balm
Family: Lamiaceae
Origin: Mediterranean region and Southern Europe

Use and Benefits: It has been used to relieve tension and anxiety, enhance appetite, promote sleep, relieve pain and discomfort associated with indigestion, such as gas, bloating, and colic, since the Middle Ages.

26. Stiff Goldenrod

Scientific name: Oligoneuron rigidum
Common names: rigid goldenrod and prairie goldenrod
Family: aster family
Origin: Canada and the United States.

Use and Benefits: The leaves and blooms work as antibacterial, astringent, and the bleeding stops. It's been used for a long time to treat many types of hemorrhages. Native Americans often crushed the blossoms to form a lotion and applied them to bee stings.

27. Red Clover

Scientific name: Trifolium pratense
Common names: red clover
Family: Fabaceae
Origin: Europe, Western Asia, and Northwest Africa

Use and Benefits: It's been used for centuries to cure whooping cough, cancer, respiratory disorders, and skin inflammation like psoriasis and dermatitis, as well as to "purify" the blood, enhance circulation, and aid menopause and heart health.

28. Coltsfoot

Scientific name: Tussilago farfara
Common names: bulls foot, British tobacco, coughwort, butterbur, horse hoof, flower velure
Family: Asteraceae
Origin: endemic to a number of European and Asian regions

Use and Benefits: For thousands of years, people have utilized this dandelion-like plant medicinally all throughout the globe. Cough and asthma were treated with it according to Pedanius Dioscorides, a Greek physician and pharmacologist who flourished from 40 to 90 AD. It was also known by other names, such as and. Cough, whooping cough, bronchitis, and other respiratory illnesses were treated using its leaves. For pleurisy, flu, inflammation, sore throat, diarrhea, fever, and indigestion, mashed leaves were used in infusions and tonics. Externally, crushed leaves and petals were used for skin problems, bug bites, burns, inflammation, sores, and skin ulcers, among other things.

29. Sweetflag

Scientific name: Acorus calamus
Common names: sweet sedge, calamus and myrtle flag
Family: Acoraceae

Origin: Southern Asia

Use and Benefits: Flatulence, colds, heart disease, intestinal issues, colic, menstrual problems, dropsy, headache, spasms, toothache, and swelling have all been treated with the root. Externally, it has been used to cure skin eruptions, rheumatoid discomfort, and arthritis.

30. Lobelia

Scientific name: Lobelia
Common names: lobelias
Family: Campanulaceae
Origin: Mostly in tropical and warm temperate climates

Use and Benefits: Lobelia has long been utilized by Native Americans to treat pulmonary and muscle ailments, as well as a purgative. The plant was used in Appalachian traditional medicine to treat asthma.

31. Ginkgo Biloba

Scientific name: Ginkgo biloba
Common names: gingko or ginkgo, maidenhair tree
Family: Ginkgoaceae
Origin: China

Use and Benefits: Because of its beneficial properties as a circulatory aid, it is most typically used to treat disorientation, memory loss, depression, tinnitus, headache, high blood pressure, dementia, Alzheimer's Disease, and vertigo in the elderly. It's also been shown to help with circulation, ADHD, high blood pressure, cramping, and as an antioxidant.

32. Yellow Dock

Scientific name: Rumex crispus
Common names: curled dock, curly dock, sour dock, and narrow dock
Family: Buckwheat family
Origin: Europe and Western Asia

Use and Benefits: Different tribes across North America employed the leaves and roots to treat constipation, blood purification, ringworm, and stomach problems. It was applied externally to treat joint discomfort, itching, small blisters, diaper rash, or other skin problems.

33. Lemon Verbena

Scientific name: Aloysia citrodora
Common names: lemon beebrush
Family: Verbenaceae
Origin: South American native

Use and Benefits: The leaves of this perennial shrub are used to lend a lemon flavor to a variety of foods and drinks. It's frequently administered as an antioxidant, and it can safeguard against oxidative damage while also reducing the indications of muscle damage.

34. Slippery Elm

Scientific name: Ulmus rubra
Common names: moose elm, red elm, soft elm, gray elm, and Indian elm
Family: Ulmaceae
Origin: Eastern North American native

Use and Benefits: Digestive problems, gastrointestinal issues, sore throats, gout, arthritis, stomach aches, intestinal worms, bronchitis, and other lung irritations were among the conditions treated.

35. Blue Spruce

Scientific name: Picea pungens
Common names: white spruce, green spruce, Colorado blue spruce or Colorado spruce
Family: Pinaceae
Origin: North American native

Use and Benefits: There are a number of medical and therapeutic uses for black spruce. You may improve your immune system by eating spruce, which is a great source of vitamin C. Spruce is an excellent expectorant because of its affinity for the lungs. Spruce may be used as a steam cleaner for this purpose.

36. Goldenrod

Scientific name: Solidago Virgaurea or Solidago Canadensis
Common names: goldenrods
Family: Asteraceae
Origin: North American

Use and Benefits: Goldenrod has traditionally been used as a topical treatment for wounds. Tuberculosis, diabetes, liver enlargement, gout, hemorrhoids, internal bleeding, asthma, kidney stones, arthritis, flu, colds, bladder, and urinary inflammation, allergies, sore throat, laryngitis, mouth ulcers, cuts, and abrasions have all been treated with it. It can combat infection since it contains both antibacterial and anti-inflammatory properties.

37. Mayapple

Scientific name: Podophyllum peltatum
Common names: American mandrake, ground lemon, ducks foot, Indian apple, love apple, hog apple, racoon berry
Family: Berberidaceae
Origin: eastern North America

Use and Benefits: The roots of these plants were utilized as a laxative to cure worms and improve liver function, indicating that healers understood what they were doing. Snakebite, warts, and other skin diseases were treated with it externally. Only professional herbalists should use this herb because of its toxicity.

38. Cinnamon Bark

Scientific name: Cinnamomum cassia
Common names: Chinese cinnamon or Chinese cassia
Family: Lauraceae
Origin: Southeast Asian in origin

Use and Benefits: It has a long history of medicinal usage in many cultures and has been used to improve cognitive performance and memory, cure colds, rheumatism, diarrhea, diabetes, toothaches, aid digestion, and ease some menstruation issues throughout the years. Because it includes substantial antioxidant potential, drinking tea brewed from Sri Lanka cinnamon bark on a regular basis is regarded to be helpful to oxidative stress-related disorders.

39. Wild Rose

Scientific name: Rosa canina
Common names: hip fruit, sweetbriar, brier hip, briar rose, dogberry, and witch's brier
Family: Rosaceae
Origin: Europe, northwest Africa, and western Asia

Use and Benefits: The Wild Rose's mature fruit is high in Vitamin C, which is effective for cold prevention and treatment. Hip tea is a light diuretic that also stimulates the kidneys and bladder. Inflammation, bladder, stress, infection, gout, digestion, rheumatism, fever, and immunological, reproductive, circulatory, and neurological system support are among the other uses.

40. Fennel

Scientific name: Foeniculum Vulgare
Common names: fennel
Family: Apiaceae
Origin: The Mediterranean coasts

Use and Benefits: Fennel was used as a digestive aid in Puritan folk medicine. The leaves, roots, and seeds of fennel are harmless and edible, but the essential oil collected from the seeds could be hazardous, even in little amounts. It's been used for years for a digestive aid, flatulence cure, appetite stimulant, and to help nursing women produce more breast milk. Teas and tonics made from the leaves and seeds were used to cure stomach pains, newborn colic, coughs, colds, respiratory issues, and constipation.

41. American Licorice

Scientific name: Glycyrrhiza lepidota pursh
Common names: wild licorice
Family: Fabaceae
Origin: Indigenous to Canada and the Northwest United States (Texas California)

Use and Benefits: One of the world's oldest herbal treatments is the root of the U.S. licorice plant. Teas, supplements, tinctures, medications, and powders all include this root, which has long been used to treat a wide range of medical ailments. It is often used to treat viral infections, cough, heartburn, hot flashes, and acid reflux. Sore throats and tough skin diseases may also be alleviated by using them. Treat peptic ulcers and prevent cavities. Menopause symptoms, high blood sugar, and skin conditions may all be alleviated by using this supplement.

42. Chickweed

Scientific name: Stellaria pubera & Stellaria media
Common names: star chickweed, common chickweeds, and mouse-ear chickweed
Family: Caryophyllaceae
Origin: Eurasia

Use and Benefits: It may be found all throughout North America, from Alaska's Brooks Range to Mexico. The whole plant, which is rich in many nutrients, has been used to treat diarrhea, cough, cystitis, and renal and urinary tract issues, as well as as an antihistamine, astringent, expectorant, and diuretic. Rheumatic aches, wounds, ulcers, roseola, itchy skin disorders, cuts, small burns, eczema, and rashes have all been treated using poultices on the outside.

43. Western Skunk Cabbage

Scientific name: Lysichiton americanus
Common names: swamp lantern and yellow skunk cabbage
Family: Araceae
Origin: Pacific Northwest

Use and Benefits: The herb was utilized by Native Americans to treat burns and injuries, as well as sores and swelling.

44. Burdock

Scientific name: Arctium lappa
Common names: cocklebur & bardana
Family: Asteraceae
Origin: It's believed to have come from Eurasia.

Use and Benefits: Vegetarians all around the globe have long consumed the roots of this plant, which may also be used medicinally for a variety of gastrointestinal and respiratory conditions. Root and leaf crushing were used to alleviate rheumatism in Native Americans, as well as to treat skin conditions like sores. Roots of the plant were used by the Iroquois to improve circulation and cleanse the blood.

45. Guarana

Scientific name: Paullinia cupana
Common names: Guaraná
Family: Sapindaceae
Origin: The Amazon Basin

Use and Benefits: It has caffeine in it and is commonly taken as a stimulant. Over time, it's been used to treat headaches, moderate depression, persistent diarrhea, weariness, arthritis, and urinary tract irritation, among other things. It stimulates the neurological system, promotes energy, enhances metabolism, and reduces appetite in the same way that coffee does. It was also used as an aphrodisiac and to combat malaria and dysentery in the past.

46. Cardinal Flower

Scientific name: Lobelia cardinalis
Common names: cardinal flower
Family: Campanulaceae
Origin: From southern Canada to the east and southern parts of the United States as well as Mexico and Central America.

Use and Benefits: Native Americans have used the root to treat worms, epilepsy, typhoid fever, cramps, and syphilis, among other things. It is still widely used today. For bronchial problems, colds, croup, and nosebleeds, as well as fever and rheumatoid arthritis, leaf tea was an effective remedy. People have employed a root poultice on difficult-to-heal wounds and on their heads to alleviate migraine headache discomfort.

47. Buck Brush

Scientific name: Ceanothus cuneatus
Common names: buckbrush or wedgeleaf ceanothus

Family: Rhamnaceae -Buckthorn Family

Origin: California, Oregon, and northern Baja California are home to this species.

Use and Benefits: Inflammation of the tonsils, non-fibrous cysts, enlarged lymph nodes, non-enlarged spleen, menstrual bleeding, nosebleeds, and ulcers may all be treated with it, as well as anxiety and anxiousness. Sores, burn wounds, and other wounds were treated using poultices.

48. Yellow Root

Scientific name: Xanthorhiza simplicissima
Common names: goldenseal
Family: Ranunculaceae
Origin: eastern United States.

Use and Benefits: While Yellow Root is deadly in massive doses, Native Americans utilized it to make tea for mouth problems, gastrointestinal disorders, and stomach aches, as well as to cure sores, skin disorders, and swelling externally. It has also been discovered to aid in the reduction of blood pressure and the maintenance of liver health.

49. Hibiscus

Scientific name: Hibiscus
Common names: common hibiscus and China rose
Family: Malvaceae
Origin: warm temperate, subtropical, and tropical climates all throughout the world.

Use and Benefits: Hibiscus is a flowering plant that is used to treat respiratory and skin ailments. Internally for gastrointestinal issues and topically as an emollient. Constipation, skin disorders, hemorrhoids, menstrual cramps, wounds, headache, TB, PMS, stomach problems, along with alleviating labor pains and regulating blood pressure, have all been treated with it over the years.

BOOK 20

HERBAL MEDICINES & PLANT REMEDIES. - VOLUME 4

1. Cat's Claw

Scientific name: Uncaria tomentosa
Common names: cat's nail
Family: Rubiaceae
Origin: Asia and South America are the two continents where this species is found.

Use and Benefits: It's been used as a basic health tonic, anti-inflammatory agent, contraceptive, urinary and gastrointestinal tract issues, diarrhea, rheumatic illnesses, respiratory difficulties, acne, and diabetes for more than two millennia. Current research suggests it may benefit the immune system, aid in the treatment of diabetes, Aids, chronic fatigue syndrome, PMS, prostate issues, and cancer, among other things.

2. American Mistletoe

Scientific name: Rhododendron leucippus
Common names: guy American, eastern mistletoe, mistletoe, guy de chine, rhododendron flavescent, murage americano
Family: Santalike
Origin: Inhabitants of the United States (Florida, New Mexico, Illinois)

Use and Benefits: A valuable plant with multiple applications, American mistletoe dates back to at least the early 1920s. Everything on this plant is therapeutic, including the leaf, stem, flower, and fruit. To treat constipation and low blood pressure, American mistletoe has compounds that impact the muscles.

3. Mountain Hemlock

Scientific name: Tsuga mertensiana
Common names: mountain hemlock
Family: Pinaceae
Origin: native to North America's west coast

Use and Benefits: The bark is diuretic, diaphoretic, and astringent. A tea produced from the bark or twigs can assist with influenza, colds, kidney and bladder disorders, and it also works well as an enema for diarrhea.

4. Cloves

Scientific name: Syzygium aromaticum
Common names: cengkih, clove, and chengkeh
Family: Myrtaceae
Origin: Indonesian native

Use and Benefits: It is used as a spice as well as in medicine. Toothache, cough, poor breath, gum troubles, skin infection, indigestion, nausea, flatulence, and heartburn are some of the conditions that may be treated with this medicine. Antioxidant properties are also present.

5. Greenbriar

Scientific name: Smilax nona-nox
Common names: bullbriar, prickly-ivy, horsebriar, catbriar
Family: Smilacaceae
Origin: native to the eastern United States

Use and Benefits: Its root has long been employed as a diuretic, in the therapy of dropsy, urinary problems, and as a blood cleanser by flowering plants, most of which are thorny and/or woody. Tea brewed from the roots has long been utilized to aid in the removal of afterbirth and so as a tonic for rheumatism and stomach disorders.

6. Chasteberry

Scientific name: Vitex agnus
Common names: chaste tree, vitex, Abraham's balm, chasteberry
Family: Lamiaceae
Origin: Mediterranean indigenous

Use and Benefits: The fruit has been used for centuries to help relieve menstruation cramps and boost breast milk supply. It was purportedly employed by priests in the Medieval Era to reduce sexual desire and maintain chastity, thus the name. It's also referred to as vitex, chaste tree berry, and monk's pepper. The herb, on the other hand, seems to have no effect on sexual desire.

7. Boswellia

Scientific name: Boswellia serrata
Common names: Boswellia serrata, Boswellia, Boswellia, Boswellia
Family: Burseraceae
Origin: India, Arabs, and Africa are all home to this species.

Use and Benefits: Boswellia is a prevalent tree in Ayurveda, the Indian system of medicine. Brain damage, rheumatoid arthritis, osteoarthritis, bursitis, joint pain, and swelling of tendons may all be treated with Boswellia, which is taken orally as an anti-inflammatory agent (tendonitis). For ulcerative colitis, inflammation of the colon, Crohn's disease, and stomach discomfort, it is also given by mouth. Menstrual cramps and discomfort, hives, sore throat, syphilis, and asthma are only a few of the conditions for which it is utilized. Menstrual flow is aided by the usage of Boswellia as a stimulant and to improve urine flow. Substances found in the resin of Boswellia may reduce inflammation and boost the immune system.

8. Wild Carrot

Scientific name: Daucus carota
Common names: bishop's lace, bird's nest, and Queen Anne's lace
Family: Apiaceae
Origin: Native to Europe's temperate zones and southwest Asia

Use and Benefits: Digestive issues, kidney and bladder ailments, dropsy, flatulence, and menstruation problems are among the traditional uses.

9. Spearmint

Scientific name: Mentha spicata
Common names: spearmint, garden mint, spearmint or menthol mint
Family: mint family
Origin: Europe and southwest Asia

Use and Benefits: The flavor of a medicinal herb tea brewed from fresh and dried leaves is pleasant and refreshing. Fever, bronchitis, common cold, headache, nasal congestion, indigestion, morning and motion sickness, nausea, and painful menstruation have all been treated with it. It has been used externally to treat injuries, stiffness, muscle discomfort, and rheumatism.

10. Wild Cherry

Scientific name: Prunus avium
Common names: sweet cherry, wild cherry, or bird cherry
Family: Rosaceae
Origin: Europe, Maghreb, Anatolia, and West Asia

Use and Benefits: The fruit and bark were used to create medicine across Europe, Anatolia, the Maghreb, and Western Asia. For colds, lung inflammation, and other lung issues, some individuals take wild cherry by mouth.

11.Pennyroyal

Scientific name: Mentha pulegium
Common names: mosquito plant, tickweed, mock pennyroyal, fleabane, and stinking balm
Family: Mint family
Origin: Northern Africa, Middle East and Europe

Use and Benefits: It was employed to get rid of pests like snakes. Despite the fact that it is toxic, Native Americans used American Pennyroyal to treat fever, stomach pains, watery eyes, itching, and to induce menstrual flow. They mashed the leaves and put them on the epidermis as an insect repellent on the outside.

12. Devil's Claw

Scientific name: Harpagophytum procumbens
Common names: harpagon, grapple plant, devil's club, and wood spider
Family: Pedaliaceae
Origin: Southern African native

Use and Benefits: It was utilized as a numbing agent and to cure rheumatoid arthritis, fever, skin disorders, and diseases affecting the pancreas, gallbladder, kidneys, and stomach for centuries by indigenous people in that nation. Later, it was introduced to Europe, where it was largely used to aid digestion and cure arthritis. Swelling, gout, arthritis, back pain, headaches, diarrhea, constipation, skin disorders, sores, and hunger stimulation are all treated with the roots and tubers. Because it is known to produce uterine contractions, women who are or could be pregnant should avoid using the devil's claw.

13. Indian Paintbrush

Scientific name: Castilleja
Common names: Prairie-fire
Family: Orobanchaceae
Origin: native to the Americas' west coast, from Alaska to the Andes

Use and Benefits: Indian Paintbrush is now used by the Chippewa Indians as a rheumatism treatment as well as a hair glossing bath rinse.

14. American Ginseng

Scientific name: Panax quinquefolius
Common names: baie rouge, anchi ginseng, ginseng, and Canadian ginseng
Family: Ivy
Origin: a plant found only in deciduous woodlands

Use and Benefits: The adaptogen properties of American ginseng are well accepted. There is a family of drugs known as "adaptogens" that are thought to increase the body's resilience to environmental, physical, and emotional stresses, as well as psychological stress. Ginsenosides, a group of compounds found in American ginseng, have been shown to reduce blood sugar and insulin levels. Iron deficiency, indigestion, flu and colds may all be treated with this supplement.

15. Elder

Scientific name: Sambucus
Common names: elderberry, elder, black elder, European elderberry, European elder,
Family: Adoxaceae
Origin: Europe and North America

Use and Benefits: Elders have traditionally been utilized in medicinal cures and as a portion of food when they ripen. The berries were used to make syrup, as well as alcoholic beverages and wine when combined with water in a fruit drink. To cure constipation and flu, traditional herbal medicine used berries and dried blossoms in teas and tonics. To sweat off pollutants, the Delaware and Cherokee brewed tea of the dried blossoms.

16. Cotton

Scientific name: Gossypium herbaceum
Common names: upland cotton
Family: Malvaceae
Origin: Tropical and subtropical plants that may be found in tropical and subtropical locations all over the globe, including the Africa, Americas, and India.

Use and Benefits: Urinary difficulties have been treated using roots, leaves, and seeds to help with uterine contractions after delivery, heavy bleeding throughout menstruation, wound and burn healing, dysentery, and diarrhea. To treat childbirth pains, Koasati tribes and Alabama brewed tea from the plant's roots.

17. Shave-grass

Scientific name: Equisetuma arvense
Common names: scouring rush horsetail, ough horsetail, and scouring rush
Family: Equisetaceae
Origin: areas of North America's southeast

Use and Benefits: Shavegrass has been used as a folk cure for kidney and bladder problems, arthritis, bleeding ulcers, TB, wound treatment, and bleeding control in several cultures, making it a general treatment for hemorrhoids and nosebleeds.

18. Feverwort

Scientific name: Triosteum Perfoliatum
Common names: horse gentian, wild coffee, fever-root, and tinker's weed
Family: Asteraceae
Origin: Canada and the Eastern United States are home to this species.

Use and Benefits: It's been used to treat diarrhea, nausea, flu, joint stiffness, itching welts, back discomfort, and pleurisy for many years. To treat fever, the Cherokee consumed its decoction. Feverwort is another name for Boneset.

19. Beeswax

Scientific name: Cera alba
Common names: Apis mel, apic cerana, Apis mellifica, Apis mellifera, bees wax
Family: Apidae

Use and Benefits: Beeswax is created from the honeycombs of honeybees and other bees. Bees travel 150,000 miles and consume 8 times as much nectar to produce one lb. of beeswax. Beeswax is used in medicine to decrease cholesterol and alleviate discomfort. There are several more uses, including the treatment of hiccups, hiccups, and swelling (inflammation). Beeswax has a slight antiinflammatory (anti-swelling) action. In addition, there is some indication that it may protect the intestines.

20. Schisandra

Scientific name: Magnoliav vine
Common names: five-flavor-fruit or magnolia berry
Family: Schisandraceae
Origin: Northern China's woodlands

Use and Benefits: It is a tonic plant that can boost mood, strengthen the liver, increase sexual function, heal skin irritations, respiratory disorders, cough, weariness, and antioxidant properties. It has also been shown in laboratory trials to improve blood pressure, cognitive efficiency, nervous system function, endurance, and strength.

21. Coneflower

Scientific name: Echinacea
Common names: coneflowers
Family: Asteraceae
Origin: North America's east and center

Use and Benefits: In traditional medicine, Echinacea purpurea is employed. Despite the fact that Echinacea medications are widely promoted as dietary supplements, there is little scientific proof that they are beneficial or safe for enhancing health or curing any condition.

22. Green Tea

Scientific name: Camellia Sinensis
Common names: Green Tea
Family: Theaceae
Origin: China

Use and Benefits: It has been used as a stimulant and a diuretic in Thailand, Japan, China, and India, where it has been used to control bleeding, treat wounds, enhance cardiovascular health, treat flatulence, stimulate digestion, manage blood sugar, and boost brain processes. It's now being used to treat cancer, inflammatory bowel disease, diabetes and liver disease, as well as decrease cholesterol and encourage weight loss. It may also help with inflammatory conditions, including arthritis and the treatment of colds and flu.

23. Mugwort

Scientific name: Artemisia
Common names: St. John's plant
Family: Daisy family
Origin: Eastern Asia and Europe

Use and Benefits: For hundreds of years, both the roots and leaves have been used to relieve gas and bloating, uterine stimulant, digestive stimulant, to induce delayed menstruation, relaxation, and as a moderate sedative.

24. Grapefruit

Scientific name: Citrus maxima
Common names: pomelo
Family: Rutaceae
Origin: Asia

Use and Benefits: It's a subtropical citrus tree with a bitter fruit that's growing all over the world. Its seeds, flesh, and inner skin have been proven to be effective in preventing both fungal and bacterial illnesses, making it a wonderful source of numerous nutrients that assist in a balanced diet. Grapefruit is a strong source of vitamin C, and it also includes antioxidants that have been shown to decrease cholesterol, inhibit kidney stones, and fight against colon cancer. Grapefruit peel contains vitamins and minerals that are used to treat stomach problems.

25. Dong Quai

Scientific name: Angelica sinensis

Common names: dang gui, Chinese angelica, tang kuei, and the female ginseng

Family: Cornaceae

Origin: Japan, China, and Korea are all home to this species.

Use and Benefits: Although there is inadequate proof that it has any medical benefit, the dried root of A. sinensis is commonly utilized in traditional Chinese medicine.

26. Yerba Mate

Scientific name: Ilex paraguariensis

Common names: Erva Mate

Family: Aquifoliaceae

Origin: South American native

Use and Benefits: It's been used for a long time as a herbal remedy for everything from boosting immunity and cleansing the blood to reducing stress and combating insomnia.

27. James' Buckwheat

Scientific name: Eriogonum jamesii

Common names: antelope sage and James' buckwheat

Family: Polygonaceae

Origin: southwest United States

Use and Benefits: This herb was employed as a contraceptive by several indigenous North American Indian cultures. During menstruation, the woman should drink 1 cup of root decoction. To ease the agony of childbirth, a decoction of an entire plant was consumed.

28. Feverfew

Scientific name: Tanacetum Parthenium

Common names: feverfew, Pyrethrum parthenium and Chrysanthemum parthenium

Family: Asteraceae

Origin: Eurasia's native species

Use and Benefits: The term "feverfew" is derived from the Latin word febrifugia, which means "fever reliever," and it has been used to cure headaches, particularly arthritis, migraines, and digestive issues.

Menstrual abnormalities, labor difficulties, skin diseases, stomach pains, and asthma have all been treated with it. Feverfew may interfere with the effects of several prescription and nonprescription medications, so ask your doctor before taking it. Long-term usage followed by rapid discontinuation might result in a withdrawal syndrome characterized by rebound headaches, muscle and joint pains, and other symptoms. People who are allergic to the components of feverfew may experience adverse responses, and it must not be taken by pregnant women.

29. Goldenseal

Scientific name: Hydrastis Canadensis
Common names: yellow root, puccoon, orange root, wild Curcuma and ground raspberry
Family: Ranunculaceae
Origin: southeastern Canada and the northeastern United States.

Use and Benefits: Traditionally, it was used by Native Americans to cure skin disorders, digestive problems, liver conditions, diarrhea, as a stimulant, and for eye irritations. The Cherokee have also been reported to use bear fat to pound the big rootstock and apply it on their body as a mosquito repellant.

30. Poke

Scientific name: Phytolacca americana
Common names: redweed, American nightshade, inkberry, pokeweed, pigeon berry, Pocan bush
Family: Phytolaccaceae
Origin: eastern United States

Use and Benefits: It is being used to treat diphtheria, syphilis, cancer, intestinal worms, asthma, cramps, and stomach ulcers, as well as inflammation and purgatives. Skin diseases, arthritis, abscesses, rheumatism, swelling, discomfort, sprains, and hemorrhoids were all treated with poultices and washes applied externally. Because this herb is dangerous, it should only be used by people who have received expert training.

31. Kola Nut

Scientific name: Cola nitida
Common names: cola, kola, kola nut, and bitter kola
Family: Malvaceae
Origin: Africa's tropical rainforests

Use and Benefits: It's been used to cure asthma, whooping cough, bronchial difficulties, anxiety, depression, improve energy, and reduce hunger for therapeutic purposes. In the 1800s, a Georgia pharmacist combined kola and coca extracts with sugar, other components, and effervescent water to create the very first cola soft drink, Coca-Cola. Kola nut is still utilized as a complementary medicine today, owing to its antidepressant qualities

32. Savory

Scientific name: Satureja
Common names: summer savory, mountain savory, and winter savory
Family: Mint family
Origin: North Africa, south and southeast Europe

Use and Benefits: It also has a variety of medical applications, including assisting the digestive system and treating gas, diarrhea, cough, and colic.

33. Sassafras

Scientific name: Sassafras albidum
Common names: sassafras
Family: Lauraceae
Origin: From Maine to Ontario and south to Florida and Texas, this plant is indigenous to eastern North America.

Use and Benefits: Measles, chickenpox, common cold, flu, temperature, as a blood cleanser, and as a cure have all been treated with it over the years.

34. Maca

Scientific name: Lepidium meyenii
Common names: maca-maca, ayak chichira, maino, and ayak willku
Family: Ginseng family
Origin: Peru's and Bolivia's high Andes

Use and Benefits: Though not a Ginseng, Peruvian Ginseng is also known as "Peruvian Ginseng" due to its reputation for enhancing stamina, libido, vitality, and sexual function. It is also reported to be helpful in the treatment of lethargy, infertility, menopause symptoms, and cancer.

35. Yellow Spined Thistle

Scientific name: Cirsium ochrocentrum
Common names: yellow spined thistle
Family: Asteraceae
Origin: native to the mid-Atlantic region of the United States

Use and Benefits: It was utilized by the Zuni nation for a variety of purposes, including contraception, syphilis treatment, and diabetic treatment. The herb was also used as a wash for ulcers, burns, and other skin ailments by the Kiowa.

36. Pleurisy Root

Scientific name: Asclepias tuberosa
Common names: butterfly weed, tuber root, flux root, Canada root, swallow-wort, white root
Family: Apocynaceae
Origin: Eastern North American native

Use and Benefits: Because of its capacity to reduce inflammation, it has traditionally been proven to be a helpful treatment for a variety of respiratory illnesses. Cough, lung inflammation, pneumonia, uterine diseases, pain, bronchitis, spasms, flu, and promoting sweating have all been treated with it.

37. Black Raspberry

Scientific name: Rubus occidentalis
Common names: blackcap, blackberry, dewberry, black raspberry
Family: Rosaceae
Origin: Eastern North American native

Use and Benefits: Raspberry is a kind of fruit. The berry (fruit) is a well-known snack item. Along with the leaves, the berries are used to produce medicines. The black raspberry may be used to alleviate stomach cramps and to avert cancer. Preventing DNA mutations and cutting off blood flow to tumors may help prevent cancer. Black raspberry includes compounds that may do this.

38. Glucomannan

Use and Benefits: It is a nutritional fiber derived from the root of a Konjac Plant that has long been used in Asian traditional meals like noodles and tofu. Constipation, Type 2 diabetes, cholesterol reduction, and weight loss are all established medical uses. It is not advised for use by women who are pregnant or breastfeeding.

39. Star Grass

Scientific name: Hypoxis
Common names: African potato and African star grass
Family: Hypoxidaceae
Origin: South African native

Use and Benefits: Traditional healers have long employed the roots, which come in a variety of species, to cure bladder infections, cardiac weakness, internal malignancies, and neurological diseases.

40. Yerba Sant

Scientific name: Yerba santa
Common names: bear's weed, Eriodictyon, and consumptive's weed
Family: Boraginaceae
Origin: California

Use and Benefits: Teas were used to cure coughs, colds, tuberculosis, loosen phlegm, asthma, and long-term swelling of the lungs' airways. It was also used to treat asthma.

41. Calamus Root

Scientific name: Acorus calamus
Common names: sway, muskrat root, & sweet flag
Family: Acoraceae
Origin: indigenous to Asia,

Use and Benefits: Calamus is thought to contain chemicals that relax muscles and induce sleep. They may also reduce inflammation, destroy cancer cells and pest problems.

42. Stevia

Scientific name: Stevia rebaudiana
Common names: sugarleaf and sweetleaf
Family: Asteraceae
Origin: West-to-South America

Use and Benefits: It has long been used to treat heartburn, overweight, flatulence, diabetes, and hypertension, as well as a sweetener.

43. Wild Garlic

Scientific name: Allium sativum
Common names: buckrams, cowleek, broad-leaved garlic, cowlic, wood garlic
Family: Amaryllidaceae
Origin: European and Asian native

Use and Benefits: Diarrhea, colic, asthma, indigestion, bronchitis, emphysema, and lack of appetite have all been treated using leaves, blossoms, and bulbs. The juice is given externally to arthritic and rheumatic joints to help with weight loss. Garlic is also said to aid in the prevention of heart disease and cancer, as well as the reduction of cholesterol and hypertension.

44. Osha

Scientific name: Ligusticum porteri
Common names: bear root, osha root, Porter's licorice root, Colorado cough root
Family: Umbellifers
Origin: Southwest

Use and Benefits: The entire plant has been utilized for medicinal purposes, but the dense taproots are the most prized. It possesses a wide range of medical effects. Fresh and dried Osha roots were used in teas, tinctures and ingested for internal use, as well as salves and poultices for external use. It has been known for its warming effects, which have been used to treat colds and chills, as well as to improve circulation. Sore muscles, bodily aches, rheumatic, and arthritis were treated with salves and liniments.

FREQUENTLY ASKED QUESTIONS

Question: What is the definition of an herb?

Answer:

An herb is a plant used either for its culinary value, or for therapeutic purposes. Herbs are part of the major forms of treatment traditionally used in many cultures, alongside animal products.

Question: What is the correct description of herbal medicine?

Answer:

Herbal medicine can be aptly defined as the art combined with the science that makes of use plants for the sake of enhancing people's overall health. It is a mode of health enhancement that begun centuries ago; estimation being as far back as 5,000 years ago.

Question: What is the difference between herbal treatments and pharmaceuticals?

Answer:

Herbal treatments are prepared from herbs, either in their fresh form or after they have been dried. The actual treatment comes from phyto-chemicals, which are active compounds contained in the herbs.

As for pharmaceuticals, they are drugs manufactured after certain chemicals have been scientifically synthesized for the purpose of influencing particular body processes.

Another major variation of the herbal and pharmaceutical treatments is that while pharmaceuticals focus on isolation of a given active ingredient, herbalists make use of the entire spectrum of compounds in the plant. In many instances, whole plants are utilized for medicinal use; the leaves, fruits and even the roots.

Another stack difference between herbal treatments and pharmaceuticals is that there is concurrence among all modern medical practitioners regarding any particular medication; courtesy of internationally recognized regulatory bodies like the FDA, CDC, WHO and others.

On the contrary, the practice of herbal treatment is not regulated by common boards or organizations; and so certain herbalists may differ with others with regard to accepted medication dosages, acceptability of certain herbal medications, and so on.

There is also the difference in side effects. Whereas many herbal treatments are largely free of side effects, many modern medications have side effects, some of which are serious.

CONCLUSION

The practice of herbal medicine involves use of medicine extracted from different parts of plants. These medications are taken in their natural form, and they have an advantage over pharmaceuticals in that they do not ordinarily have adverse side effects.

While medicinal herbs are found in forests and other natural habitats, different ways have been devised for cultivating them. Some herbs are cultivated in domestic gardens, while others have their seeds germinated and then transplanted in forests.

Now that people of the world have generally accepted herbal medications as valuable alternative treatment, it would be great if more and more people would learn how best to do their herb harvesting, to ensure these valuable plants do not become extinct.

It would also be helpful if people learnt how to propagate and take care of their own medicinal herbs. Not only would so doing ensure safe and affordable treatments are close to home, but also that the families of herbs in the wild are not overharvested.

BONUS : VIDEO TUTORIAL

The best video tutorials chosen for you

1-Copy and paste in link or

2-Scan the QR CODE

1

https://www.youtube.com/playlist?list=PL-l73Aewt1kP8Fxba3OuFuXXP-8IBN0iV

2

Made in the USA
Las Vegas, NV
15 May 2024

89948070R00168